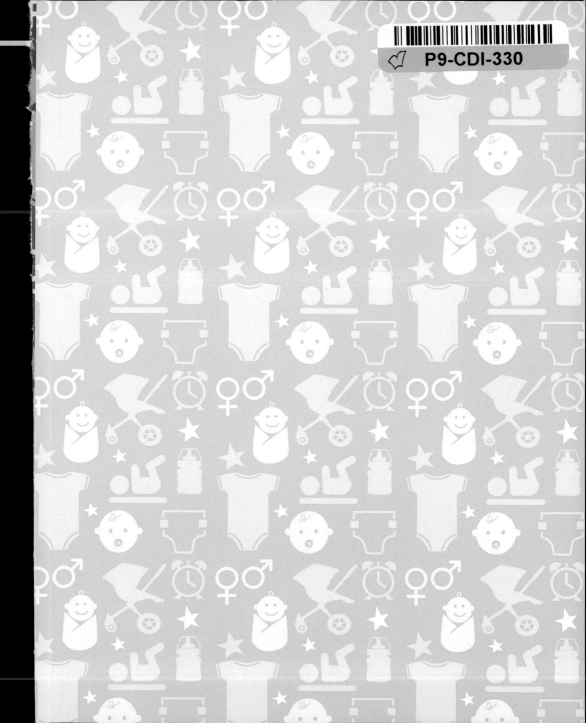

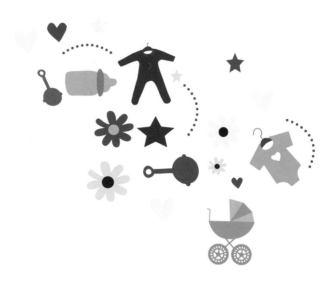

pregnancy
The Beginner's Guide

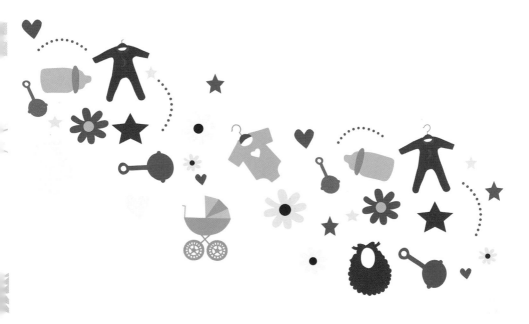

Advice from experts
- Prenatal care
- Taking care of dad
- The new arrival!

"A guide to help you as you travel through pregnancy – from conception to the birth of your baby."

pregnancy
The Beginner's Guide

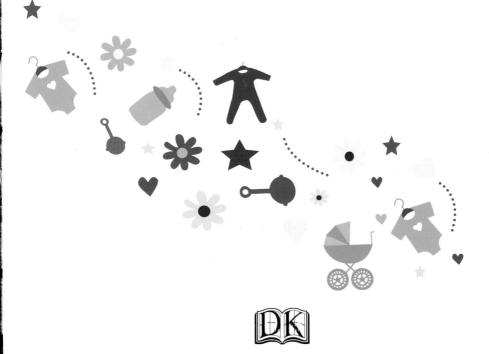

DK

DK

LONDON, NEW YORK, MUNICH, MELBOURNE, AND DELHI

DK US
US Senior Editor Shannon Beatty
US Editor Jane Perlmutter
US Consultant: Lisa Fields

DK UK
Senior Editors Christine Stroyan,
Katharine Goddard
Senior Art Editors Claire Patané, Jane Ewart
Project Editors Becky Alexander,
Joanna Edwards
US Editor Jane Perlmutter
Project Art Editors Charlotte Johnson,
Claire Shedden, Elaine Hewson, Ria Holland
Jacket Designer Rosie Levine
Illustrator Bryony Fripp
Producer, Pre-Production Sarah Isle,
Raymond Williams
Senior Producer Alex Bell
Creative Technical Support
Sonia Charbonnier
Managing Editor Penny Smith
Senior Managing Art Editor
Marianne Markham
Publisher Mary Ling
Creative Director Jane Bull
Consultant Judith Barac
Writers Shaoni Bhattacharya, Claire Cross,
Elinor Duffy, Kate Ling, and Susannah Marriott.

Every effort has been made to ensure that
the information in this book is complete and
accurate. However, neither the publisher nor the
authors are engaged in rendering professional
advice or services to the individual reader. The
contents of this book are not intended as a
substitute for consulting with your healthcare
provider. All matters regarding the health of you
and your baby require medical supervision. Neither
the publisher nor the authors shall be liable or
responsible for any loss or damage allegedly
arising from any information or suggestions
in this book.

First American Edition, 2014
Published in the United States by
DK Publishing
345 Hudson Street
New York, New York 10014

14 15 16 17 10 9 8 7 6 5 4 3 2
004-196608-Feb/14

A catalog record for this book is available
from the Library of Congress.
ISBN: 978-1-4654-1579-0

DK books are available at special discounts
when purchased in bulk for sales promotions,
premiums, fund-raising, or educational use. For
details, contact: DK Publishing Special Markets,
345 Hudson Street, New York, New York 10014
or SpecialSales@dk.com.

Published in Great Britain by
Dorling Kindersley Limited.

ISBN: 978-1-4654-1579-0

Printed and bound in China by
Leo paper products Ltd.

Discover more at **www.dk.com**

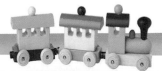

Contents

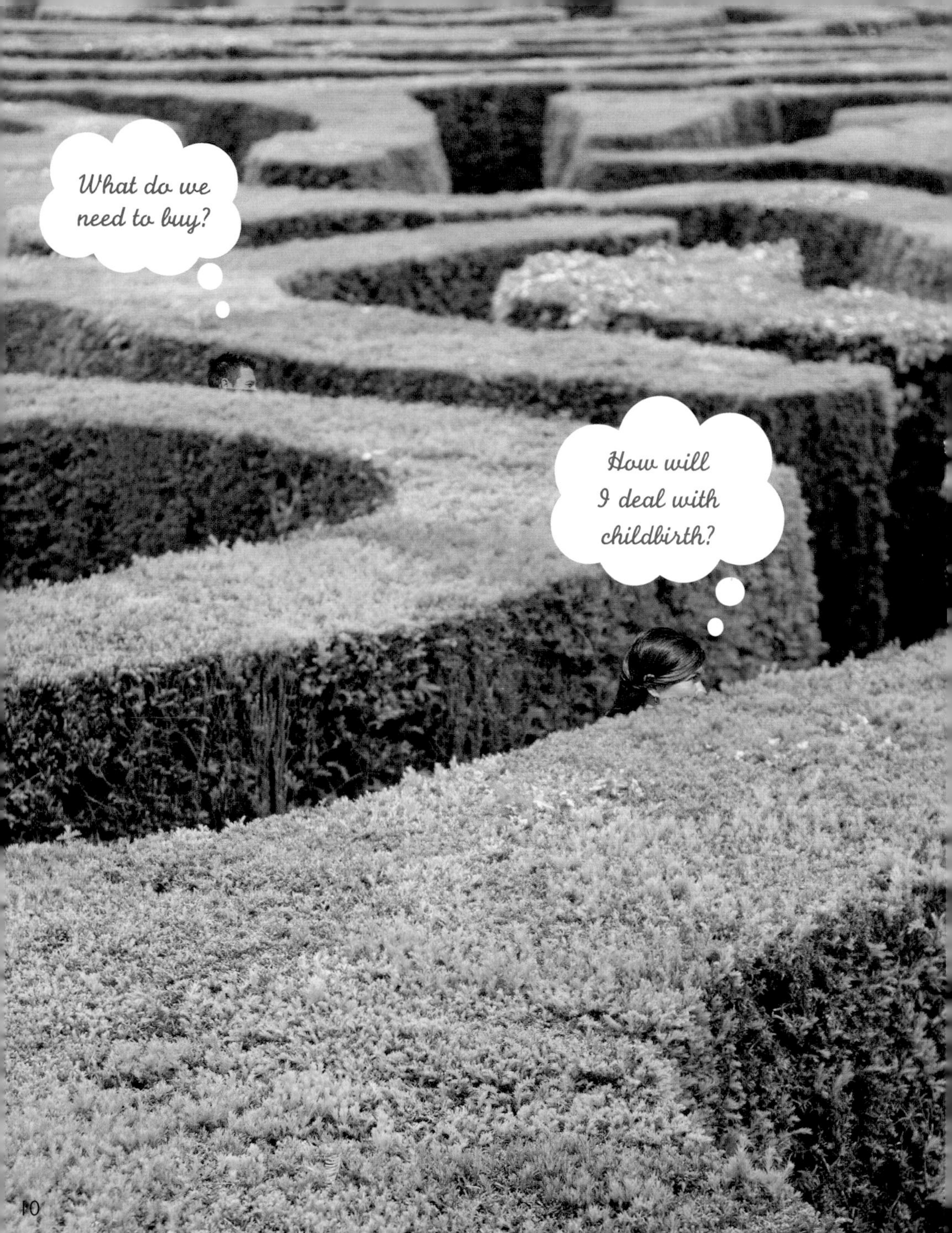
What do we need to buy?
How will I deal with childbirth?

Introduction

FINDING YOUR WAY

WELCOME TO PREGNANCY! This journey begins without you even knowing it, and ends with the happiest day of your life—the day you meet your baby. When you reach your destination one thing is for sure—your path will have changed forever, and in the best way possible.

THIS VOYAGE will take you to strange new places, such as to OB/GYN appointments and childbirth classes; you will have to get used to a different style of clothing, a change in diet, and a language you have never come across before. The journey may test your relationship with your loved ones, but will also bring you closer than ever.

PREGNANCY is an emotional roller coaster, too—your hormones run riot throughout the nine months, your body is no longer your own, and you will bounce from elation to exhaustion and back again as your life gradually shifts to accommodate enormous and unprecedented change. And then, suddenly, you have a tiny person in your care, who relies on you for everything and who will bring you more joy than you could have ever thought imaginable.

DO YOU NEED TO KNOW what to do, what to eat, and where to go? Look no further for all the answers: let *Pregnancy: The Beginner's Guide* be your constant companion as you make your way through this wonderful new world. This book will be your key to blending in, to understanding what's going on, to knowing what's ahead, and most importantly, to making the most out of every minute. You will never do this for the first time again, so don't waste a moment worrying when you could spend it understanding, marveling, and enjoying the trip of a lifetime.

You are about to embark on an epic adventure, with each step taking you closer to meeting your baby. You have 40 weeks to get acquainted with all things baby!

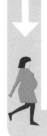

FIRST TRIMESTER

HALFWAY THERE!

FIRST OB/GYN APPOINTMENT

Yes, you are pregnant! Your hormones are busy getting ready for baby.

Weeks 5–8

FEELING PREGNANT?

Morning sickness may kick in as your body goes through amazing changes. Get plenty of rest, eat well, and take care of yourself.

SECOND TRIMESTER

Weeks 9–12

YOUR FIRST ULTRASOUND You get to see and hear your baby for the first time, and he will be checked to see that everything is well. You will also find out the estimated delivery date—when baby is due! You can get an image to take home, and may start telling people.

Weeks 17–21

20-WEEK ULTRASOUND

The sonographer will check that baby is growing well, while you get to watch your baby move around. Your baby has grown and you may find out if it's a boy or girl!

Weeks 13–16

LOOKING PREGNANT You might have a belly by now, and the secret is out! You may need to buy new clothes.

This is a travel guide to your journey from conception to delivery.

370,000 BABIES ARE BORN EVERY DAY

WEEKLY CHECKUPS

THIRD TRIMESTER

Weeks 31–35

GET ORGANIZED
Enjoy your childbirth classes, and meet lots of parents-to-be. Start packing a hospital bag so you have everything you need, ready for action.

Weeks 22–26

AND RELAX! You are probably feeling great; blooming in fact. Your skin and hair look good, and you have more energy. This could be the perfect time to take a vacation.

Weeks 36–40

COUNTING DOWN
Baby is nearly ready to be born. Good luck on your new adventure!

Weeks 27–30

PLANNING THE BIRTH Visit hospitals and birthing centers, and arrange to go to parenting classes. Talk to work about maternity leave.

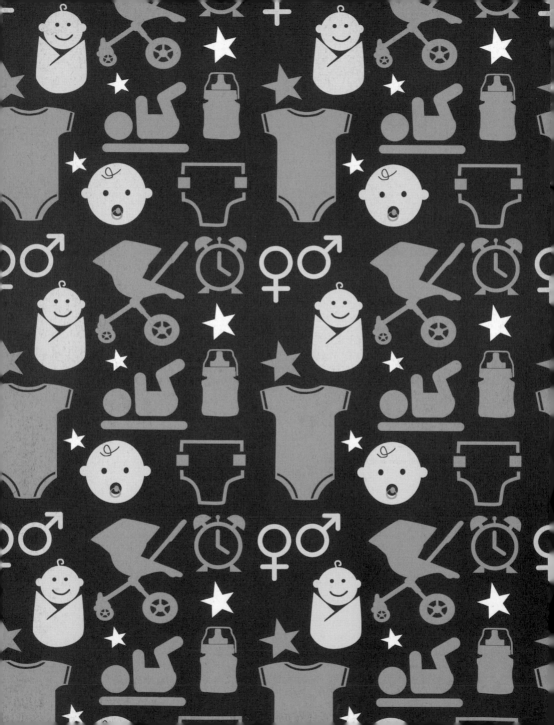

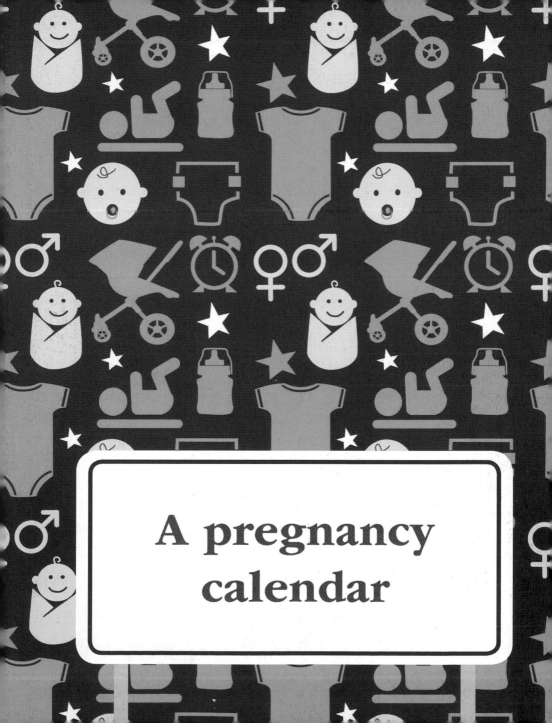

A pregnancy calendar

The journey begins

Get ready for the trip of a lifetime! Even if you don't look or feel any different, your body is busy getting ready for all the new tasks it has to perform.

✳ We have lift-off!

Levels of the female hormone estrogen, produced by your ovaries, rise rapidly during the first weeks of pregnancy. It increases blood flow to your organs, and thickens the lining of your uterus to create a welcoming environment for the implanting embryo. Working alongside the hormone progesterone, estrogen also triggers the mammary glands to swell, making your breasts feel unusually tender and heavy or tingly. Your body is getting ready for breast-feeding.

✳ It's like jet lag

Triggering many of the tell-tale signs and sensations of early pregnancy, progesterone levels also rise after conception. For the next few weeks progesterone is produced in the corpus luteum, the follicles in your ovary that burst to release the egg that was fertilized. Progesterone has a sedative effect, contributing to the unexplained exhaustion you may feel. It also relaxes your muscles and ligaments, allowing your uterus to expand. At such high levels, progesterone slows the muscle contractions that move food through your digestive system, resulting in food taking longer to be processed. This actually benefits your pregnancy—nutrients have longer to be absorbed into

x2 **BLOOD FLOW** to your uterus has already doubled. Your heart is now working hard to supply both of you!

78% **OF WOMEN** suffer from low-to-moderate prenatal psychosocial stress (anxiety).

your bloodstream—but it can also lead to indigestion, heartburn, gas, and constipation. Progesterone thickens your cervical mucus, sealing your baby safely in your uterus. It's all very clever!

✳ Testing positive

Human chorionic gonadotrophin (hCG) starts to be produced by the embryo after it implants, about a week after conception. It surges until the end of the first trimester, when it drops away steadily. This is the hormone that triggers a positive result in a pregnancy test kit. HCG prompts the corpus luteum to produce enough estrogen and progesterone to keep the embryo safely embedded and nourished until the placenta can take over production.

✳ Over the speed limit

Your metabolism speeds up after conception to support the extra demands of your organs and growing baby. Your heart pumps faster to boost blood flow to every organ, and you start to breathe more rapidly in order to deliver nutrients and oxygen to your baby. No wonder so many expectant moms feel tired!

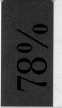

Think about booking your first doctor's appointment.

Traveling together

Pregnancy can be a nerve-wracking adventure for both partners, even if you have been planning it for a long time. Get ready for emotional swings from delight to incredulity—for both of you.

✳ PMS plus

Hormonal changes are at their most dramatic now. In fact, early pregnancy can feel like the worst case of PMS. The surge in hormones can make you moody, bloated, irritable, argumentative, and likely to burst into tears for no reason. Just being aware of this makes it more bearable, and should help your partner empathize. It's your hormones, not a personality transplant! When hormone levels even out at week 12, so should your emotions.

✳ Going long haul

You and your partner have a lot of big subjects to cover—work, money, child care—but you don't have to cover everything right now. You both have months to get used to the idea of having a baby; if you want, plan to set aside time to talk things through regularly.

✳ Your changing roles

You also don't have to decide what kind of parents to be yet, but it can help to start thinking about your backgrounds and expectations of family life. Think back to your childhoods—what do you

TOP TIP

KEEP A JOURNAL to record amusing moments, tough days, and anything else you like to help you deal with this adventure.

GOOD TO EAT
Broccoli for folic acid, vitamin A, and calcium.

remember fondly, what do you wish had been different, what would you borrow from other parents you think have done a great job.

✳ Be honest

It's best not to bluff your way through the early weeks and pretend that everything is great if it isn't. Some days pregnancy will feel like a bad idea and very few parents feel completely ready for it. The first appointment with your doctor, feeling tired, wanting to share the news, worrying about money—talk to your partner if you feel anxious.

IN PAPUA NEW GUINEA traditionally a woman does not tell her husband she is pregnant; instead she confides in family, who tells neighbors. When the husband finds out, he can't let on until the first in a series of pregnancy feasts.

✳ Expect the unexpected

Are your reactions to pregnancy what you expected? Your partner's reactions may not meet your expectations either. Becoming a parent involves finding out about your partner—like how he or she manages when faced with life changes and responsibility. You both may need to learn empathy, practice patience, and get better at talking things through. It's all good preparation for when your baby is older!

✳ Planning for your first appointment

Write down any questions you have for your first appointment. You can ask about anything that is worrying you. Your doctor, when you meet her, will be able to answer the questions and hopefully reassure you.

MONTH

1

Weeks 1–4

BABY'S JOURNEY

The sperm decides the sex of the baby, since it carries either an X or Y chromosome.

A love story

If you thought falling in love with your partner was an incredible adventure, then the romance gets really serious once egg and sperm meet. In just seven days they collide, mingle, and start a whole new person.

✳ Boy meets girl

When egg and sperm meet in your fallopian tube, they fuse to create a new cell, the zygote, in which the genetic material (DNA) they each carry mixes together. Here, your 23 chromosomes join your partner's 23 chromosomes forming a single cell with 46 chromosomes. Your baby's sex, as well as its unique looks and character, are entirely determined by this meeting and mixing of male and female DNA.

✳ The magic happens

For the first 12 hours of life the zygote remains a single cell. It starts to move down your fallopian tube, aided by the movement of tiny, hairlike structures called cilia, which propel it toward your uterus. About 30 hours into its journey, the zygote divides in two. In another 15 hours, these two cells divide to become four. And after about 72 hours have passed since fertilization, those four have divided into

Baby's progress bar: you are now 10% complete

LOADING ...

| 10% | 20% | 30% | 40% | 50% |

DID YOU KNOW?

BY DAY FOUR, the embryo contains at least 12 cells. Within a few weeks, it will grow to form a cluster of cells. Your baby already contains 46 chromosomes.

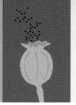

HOW BIG?
Your baby is now the size of a poppy seed.

eight cells, and the initial loose bunch of cells has become a tight ball. This process of cell division continues, over and over, until there is a cluster of around 100 cells, now called a blastocyst. At this stage, a cavity develops within the blastocyst and its cells separate to form two structures: a shell-like outer layer, and an inner cell mass.

✳ Hello baby

Around five days after conception the blastocyst finally reaches your uterus, where it slows down and rolls along the sticky uterus wall. Then, on about day six, the outer layer of cells starts to burrow into the thickened uterus lining in a process known as implantation. As it implants, the blastocyst secretes the hormone hCG, which tells your body to make enough estrogen and progesterone to support the first 12 weeks of pregnancy. After about three days implantation is complete. Once safely burrowed into the lining of your uterus, the blastocyst's inner cell mass will change and specialize in order to develop into an embryo, while its outer layer begins to form the placenta.

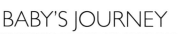

Cells at work

Deep inside your uterus an embryo is busy developing from a tiny cluster of cells. By the end of week four it has created its own beating heart.

✳ Secure luggage

After implantation, the amniotic sac starts to form from the outer cells of the blastocyte, building a protective bubble around your growing baby. The sac will fill with amniotic fluid to keep the baby warm and hydrated and act as a shock absorber. It is encircled by another protective layer, called the chorion. Tiny fingerlike "villi" reach out from here and root into the wall of your uterus, tapping into your bloodstream in order to bring nutrients and oxygen to the baby. The chorion will eventually grow into the placenta, but until this is fully formed, the embryo derives nourishment from a yolk sac, attached to it by a stalk.

✳ Ready for action

The implanted blastocyst contains an inner group of cells, each of which is programmed to create one specific aspect of the embryo. In a process called differentiation, which begins in week three, this cell mass divides into three distinct layers: the ectoderm,

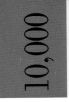

DID YOU KNOW?

PREGNANCY STARTS before you have even missed your period! Your baby is busy growing for three to four weeks before you know.

10,000

By one month, the embryo is 10,000 times larger than its initial single cell.

mesoderm, and endoderm. The cells in these layers already know whether they will become skin, skeleton, or organs, and are ready to start fulfilling these amazing and unique functions.

IN INDIAN AYURVEDIC MEDICINE, the embryo is said to be formed from the five elements that are the building blocks of all life in the universe: earth, water, fire, air, and ether. The soul enters the embryo once it is formed.

❊ Outer layer

Ectoderm cells now start to form the outer layer of your baby's body, made up of skin and hair, including the skin cells that give us pigment. So your baby's hair and eye color is being decided right now! They also form the central nervous system and the sensory organs.

❊ Middle layer

Mesoderm cells will develop into your baby's skeleton, muscles, heart, circulatory system, reproductive organs, and kidneys. Your baby's bone marrow and blood are also manufactured in this layer, alongside fat, bone, and cartilage.

❊ Inner layer

Endoderm cells make up the inner layer, and will develop into body systems including the entire digestive tract, the respiratory system, and the urinary tract, along with all the organs these systems will require to function. It's quite a substantial list, including the liver, pancreas, stomach, lungs, intestines, and bladder. There are also cells within this layer that will eventually create eggs and sperm.

Trip of a lifetime

With any long journey to a highly anticipated destination, it's always good to know roughly when you're going to get there, and pregnancy is definitely no different. You've got a lot of planning to do!

✳ Doing the math

For the sake of convenience, a baby's estimated date of delivery (EDD) is calculated as 40 weeks from the first day of the mother's last period—the specific time of conception would be far too hard to figure out. Most women with regular cycles will ovulate about two weeks after their period, so conception will usually take place around that time. This means that for the first two of the 40 weeks, the pregnancy hasn't even begun—so the baby's real time in the uterus is actually only 38 weeks. If the mathematics involved in this calculation seem boggling, help is on hand: there is a host of online calculators that, when given the date of your last period, can do the math for you. Women with irregular cycles should be aware that, for them, using this method can be somewhat hit-and-miss; the measurements taken during ultrasound dating scans are more accurate.

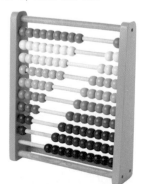

✳ Why is a due date important?

Figuring out your EDD is important for several reasons. First, it will allow the doctor to

accurately monitor your baby's growth. It will also allow you and
your partner to start thinking about future changes in your lives,
in addition to planning for maternity leave, making ultrasound
appointments, and going to childbirth classes.

✳ Patience is a virtue

The EDD might seem a lifetime away when you first discover you're
pregnant, yet many expectant moms have to wait beyond this date
for their baby to arrive. There are many reasons for this—if it is a first
pregnancy, if there is a history of post-term babies, or just if baby
isn't ready to come out yet.

✳ Ready to pop

If you reach 42 weeks, you may feel very overdue in your pregnancy
journey, but actually it's still within normal ranges. Nevertheless, most
doctors would encourage induction of labor or close monitoring after
40 weeks plus 10 days. This is because amniotic fluid levels may
begin to drop, the placenta becomes less efficient, plus the baby will
only get bigger and become more difficult to deliver. Only 5 percent
of women stay pregnant beyond 42 weeks, and in many cases this is
down to an incorrect due date prediction.

✳ Long time coming

Every day past your due date may feel like an eternity, but spare a
thought for Beulah Hunter who, in 1945, allegedly waited 375 days
for her slow-developing but perfectly healthy baby, Penny, to be
born. This remains the longest viable human pregnancy on record!

Checking that all is OK

Once you tell your doctor that you are pregnant you will make many appointments for checkups and ultrasounds. You have a whole support team to take care of you!

✳ What is the lingo?

Prenatal (meaning "before birth") care is the health care you receive while pregnant. You will have regular appointments to monitor you and your baby throughout your pregnancy. Don't worry if this is your first time in this new world; you will be given lots of information and can ask lots of questions.

✳ Who will I see?

First, you need to make an appointment with your OB/GYN, who will confirm that you are pregnant. You'll likely meet with all of the doctors in your OB/GYN's practice during your nine months, so you'll be familiar with each of them in case your usual doctor isn't on call when you go into labor. If you need specialized care you may also have appointments with a maternal fetal medicine specialist. At any appointment you have, feel free to ask questions, and write down any that occur to you between appointments. Your doctor will answer your questions and reassure you.

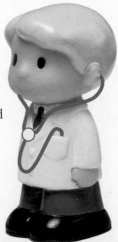

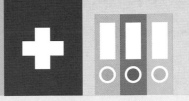

Prenatal care

✳ Check-in time

Your first meeting with a doctor at 8–12 weeks can take up to two hours and you will be asked a lot of questions including the date of your last period, whether you smoke, and if you are eating well. The goal of this is to establish how best to care for you, and to monitor how your pregnancy is progressing. You'll find out what foods and exercises to avoid and which are healthy during pregnancy. You might also be given information about recommended childbirth classes.

✳ Health checkups

You will be asked to provide a blood and urine sample to find out if you are in tip-top health. The tests will check iron levels, blood type, and look for any genetic diseases, urinary-tract infections, diabetes, and sexually transmitted diseases. If you have any medical concerns, your doctor will help you deal with them. Your baby's growth will be monitored at most appointments by measuring your belly from the top of your uterus to your pelvic bone. Your doctor may also listen to your baby's heartbeat. You will also have at least two ultrasounds (see pages 58–59 and 88–89).

✳ Final destination

Your doctor will discuss a schedule with you. Appointments will probably be monthly until 28 weeks, when they'll switch to biweekly appointments, then weekly appointments by 36 weeks. If there is any cause for concern, your doctors may refer to you a hospital for an ultrasound.

Most women only need extra calories during the last trimester —200 calories each day. That's a banana and a piece of toast.

Fruit juices, herbal teas, smoothies, and of course water make great thirst quenchers when pregnant.

What can I eat?

Forget eating for two—that's been proved wrong (sorry!). Eating a healthy, balanced diet throughout your pregnancy is best for you and your baby.

✳ Taking care of you and your baby

Your diet takes on a new significance now that you are pregnant. After all, what you eat is what your baby eats, too. Eating regular, nutritious meals and snacks will give you the energy you need for each day, alleviate nausea, and help you sleep better. There are a few foods to avoid, or cut back on (see opposite), to prevent food poisoning and the risk of E. coli, listeria, salmonella, and toxoplasmosis. Any alcohol passes to your baby, which is why the American College of Obstetricians and Gynecologists says no alcohol consumption is safe during pregnancy.

✳ Folic acid and vitamin D

Your doctor will advise you to take 400 micrograms (mcg) of folic acid throughout your first trimester; this is important since it helps prevent birth defects. You should also take 600 IU of vitamin D every day throughout your pregnancy, and continue for as long as you are breast-feeding to help your baby's bones develop healthily. If you take a multivitamin, make sure it does not contain too much vitamin A. Too much vitamin A during pregnancy can increase the risk of birth defects.

Stop!

Pâté Avoid all types, including vegetable pâtés.

Unpasteurized soft cheese This includes Camembert, Brie, soft-rind goat cheese, Roquefort, Danish blue, and Gorgonzola.

Raw eggs Risk of salmonella.

Raw or undercooked meat Especially chopped meat such as tartare or burgers.

Liver products Contain high levels of vitamin A.

Medicinal herbs Check with your doctor before taking any medicinal herbs.

Deep-sea fish Including shark, marlin, and swordfish.

Raw shellfish Cooked shellfish is usually safe.

Unpasteurized milk Risk of salmonella.

Cold meats Salami, Parma ham, chorizo, pepperoni, hot dogs, cold cuts, and processed ham due to risk of toxoplasmosis.

Caution

Caffeine Pregnant women are advised to cut back on caffeine since it can contribute to low birth weight. 200 mg a day is the advised limit, which is the equivalent of two mugs of tea or instant coffee. Chocolate also contains caffeine—dark chocolate contains about 50 mg per 50 g/2 oz bar, as does cola.

Sushi You should avoid all raw fish. See page 223.

Tuna No more than 170 g/6 oz of tuna steak and canned albacore tuna per week because tuna contains high levels of mercury.

Vegetables Must be washed to remove all traces of soil.

Commercially prepared foods Can contain listeria. Store-bought meals should be heated to a high temperature. Re-wash bagged salad greens.

Safe

Yogurt Made from pasteurized milk, including with probiotics.

Honey All types of honey.

Fruits and vegetables Wash them well before eating.

Mayonnaise If made without raw egg.

Many cheeses Hard cheeses and those made from pasteurized milk are safe.

Vegetables that contain vitamin A Spinach, for example, contains a different type of vitamin A than the one in supplements and liver.

Pasteurized cream This is safe because listeria is killed by pasteurization.

Shrimp If cooked thoroughly.

Coleslaw As long as the eggs in the mayonnaise are pasteurized, which they are in most store-bought varieties.

Peanuts Good source of protein, but not if your partner has an allergy.

Always wash your hands with soap and dry carefully before preparing food since bacteria spreads more easily on damp skin.

Choose healthy, nutritious food to refuel your body and help it to keep up with the demands of pregnancy.

A healthy balance

Whether you like to cook or prefer to buy prepared meals, making some thoughtful choices will help you to eat well. Mix in delicious superfoods to give you and your baby a nutritional boost.

❋ Food for thought

Try to eat a mix of all the food groups, including a variety of vegetables, fruit, carbohydrates, and proteins. This is not the time for low-carb diets! On an ideal day, your food should contain 50–60 percent carbohydrates, 25 percent essential fats, and 20 percent proteins. Good sources of carbohydrate include whole grains, such as whole-wheat bread, brown rice, legumes, and grains. Protein is found in legumes, nuts, eggs, dairy, meat, and fish. Essential fats come from nuts, seeds, oily fish, and eggs. Try to have carbohydrates, protein, and essential fats in every meal.

❋ Need a little extra

If you eat a varied diet then you will get the range of vitamins and nutrients that you need, but pregnancy can place extra demands on even the most foodie mom-to-be. Iron-rich foods are important during pregnancy to prevent fatigue and anemia. To help absorb iron, eat plenty of vitamin C-rich foods such as fruit or peppers.

✳ Vegetarian and gluten-free

If you know you cannot, or do not want to, eat certain foods, for example if you are diabetic or vegetarian, and are worried you may be missing essential nutrients, seek advice from a nutritionist. If you need to avoid gluten make sure you get enough energy from carbohydrates, such as sweet potatoes, quinoa, and bananas.

✳ Superfoods

You need a balanced, varied range of foods throughout your pregnancy to keep you and your baby in tip-top condition. The chart below shows a selection of the vitamins and nutrients your body can obtain from eating certain fresh foods. You may also want to refer to pages 216–221 for more information on eating well.

Vitamin A	Broccoli, carrots, sweet potatoes
Vitamin B	Broccoli, eggs, whole grains
Vitamin C	Broccoli, citrus fruits, berries, avocados
Vitamin D	Yogurt, milk, hard cheeses
Vitamin K	Spinach, dairy
Folic acid	Nuts and seeds, green leafy legumes (such as broccoli, kale, and spinach), pulses, lentils, citrus fruits, fortified cereals, avocados
Iron	Leafy green vegetables, beans and lentils, lean red meats, fortified cereals, tofu
Zinc	Nuts and seeds, beans and lentils, lean red meats
Calcium	Dairy, tofu
Omega-3/fatty acids	Oily fish, omega-3-enriched eggs, nuts
Protein	Nuts, eggs, oily fish, dairy
Potassium	Banana, avocados, sweet potatoes

I'm tired of being tired
COMMON COMPLAINTS IN EARLY PREGNANCY

WHAT TO DO

1 Fatigue
You feel exhausted and just can't do as much as you used to.

Cut down on going out in the evenings and take power naps. Listen to your body, eat healthily, and take it easy as much as possible. Fatigue should improve in the next trimester.

2 Sickness
You feel sick unless you eat a loaf of bread. You actually GET sick—a lot. It's a nightmare.

Eat little and often, and snack. Eating ginger products can help. If you can't keep anything down, see your doctor because dehydration can be dangerous in pregnancy.

3 Bloating and constipation
You have a belly full of gas and stools like rabbit droppings.

Eat lots of fiber, drink more water, and exercise daily, since this stimulates the bowel. Don't use laxatives without consulting your doctor first. Try not to strain since this causes hemorrhoids.

4 Breast changes
Your breasts are growing alarmingly and your nipples are changing color.

Get measured for maternity bras (no underwires). These will support your breasts and help ease soreness. Rub olive oil into your skin to prevent stretch marks.

5 Headaches
You're having lots of irritating minor headaches.

Drink lots of water to stave off dehydration and avoid becoming too tired. You can take acetaminophen during pregnancy, but not ibuprofen.

NEW HEALTH COMPLAINTS You may experience some, if not all, of these symptoms during your first trimester. If any are extreme, seek medical advice.

CRAVINGS could be a sign that your body needs extra minerals.

WHAT TO DO

6 Urinating all the time

You need to use the bathroom more often than usual.

This is caused by hormonal changes and the growth of the baby, and there's not much you can do. It's annoying, because it can disturb your sleep, so try to get some rest during the day.

7 Can't sleep

Tossing and turning, need the bathroom, weird taste in your mouth, crampy legs… great.

Remind yourself that you WILL be able to manage the next day and try to relax. Develop coping strategies, such as taking an afternoon nap—this is important and not a sign of laziness!

8 Cramps

Agonizing cramps in your thighs, legs, and feet.

Stretch out your leg or foot, or ask your partner to massage the cramped muscles. Some doctors say extra calcium intake can help, so ingest more milk, cheese, or bananas.

9 Food cravings

You can't stop thinking about a nice snack of grilled cheese with fries.

You are not alone in wanting favorite comfort foods such as chocolate. If you find you are craving things such as soil, charcoal, or other nonfood substances, talk to your doctor.

10 Mood swings

One minute you are laughing, the next crying.

This is normal. Sometimes just knowing that and telling those close to you is all you need to cope. Eating healthily can really help, too

Top 10

33

MONTH

1

Weeks 1–4
DAD'S SURVIVAL
GUIDE

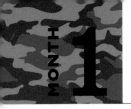

DID YOU
KNOW?

The big news!

Congratulations—you're going to be a father. From the moment the thin blue lines appear, your life changes; the positive pregnancy test signals a new phase of your life.

✳ Surprise!

It's big news. Huge. So it's hardly surprising if you experience mixed feelings; perhaps elation, pride, relief, trepidation, or downright terror. If the news is a surprise you might even be in total shock. All of this is completely natural—after all, this is probably the biggest thing that has ever happened to you. It is also the biggest thing to happen to your partner, and it is she who will be going through the most changes, so she is going to need your support, and that begins right now. Start as you mean to go on and smile, hug her, give her a kiss, and tell her this is the best news you've ever heard.

CELEBRATE YOUR amazing news with a good night out and discuss everything that's wonderful and crazy about beginning this new life.

YOUR PARTNER was born with all her eggs; half your baby is as old as her.

THE AVERAGE EJACULATION contains 40–600 million, sperm but only about 200 will be hardy enough to make it past the cervix and into the uterus.

EACH MONTH the average couple has only a 20% chance of conceiving. It's not easy!

✳ Unreal life

Initially it may all seem a bit unreal; there is no big belly, no ultrasound picture, and your partner looks the same. You may decide not to tell anyone for a few more months, which can make it all seem less tangible. You can, however, talk with your partner about the future, practicalities, and fantasize about how much fun the three of you are going to have over the rest of your lives.

✳ From tiny acorns

At this point your baby is only tiny, but she's already firmly fixed into the lining of your partner's uterus, and is busy growing. Your partner is likely experiencing very few symptoms, but she may start to have a sense that something is different, or have early nausea, and her breasts may start to grow as the pregnancy hormones start to influence her body. Your partner may start to feel more tired than usual, or she may not really notice anything different. It is time to simply let the news sink in and start to adjust to this new phase of life.

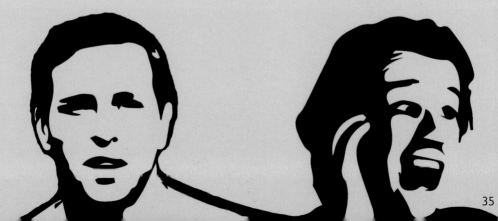

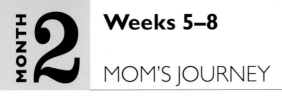
Anytime sickness

Remember how it felt to be carsick? Well, that's how it feels to have "morning sickness," which is very common during this stage of pregnancy. Sadly, for some women this nausea can occur at anytime.

✳ How are you feeling?

Many women start experiencing pregnancy symptoms around the time they miss their first period; thankfully most ease after week 12. You may experience nausea and vomiting, but other symptoms include a metallic taste in the mouth or an increase in saliva. You may have greater sensitivity to smell or food, and crave bland, filling foods, such as white bread, plain pasta, milk, and potatoes. Combined with the overwhelming exhaustion of early pregnancy, suffering from intense morning sickness can be particularly debilitating. If you can't keep any food or water down (a condition known as hyperemesis gravidarum [HG]) you need to see your doctor.

✳ What's happening inside

Morning sickness is most often attributed to rising hormones, particularly the effects of high levels of estrogen. This also contributes to your heightened sense of smell. Increased progesterone is linked to sluggish digestion, and a peak of hCG (see page 17) in month two triggers the nausea. Certain scientists explain it as an evolutionary adaptation; we instinctively choose bland foods to protect us from

DID YOU KNOW?

SIPPING WATER throughout the day can help to ease the symptoms of nausea.

GOOD TO EAT Ginger relieves nausea, stimulates the appetite, and encourages digestion.

ingesting potentially toxic plants. Bland foods are also easy to digest and the extra carbohydrates are craved when your body is saying you are tired.

✳ Take it easy

If pregnancy is making you feel tired, then listen to your body. Fatigue has been shown to worsen symptoms of morning sickness, so rest when you need to. Stay in bed a little longer in the morning if you can, rest during breaks at work rather than rushing around, and take a nap on weekends.

✳ Self-help strategies

Eating small, frequent, carbohydrate-rich snacks, such as rice cakes, oat cookies, or a slice of toast, can help to reduce morning sickness. Ginger can be extremely effective at preventing and alleviating pregnancy nausea. Most research studies recommend taking 250 mg (which is ½ tsp) of powdered ginger four times a day—you can buy this in tablets and capsules. You could also try using fresh ginger in your cooking, such as in a stir-fry, or try nibbling ginger cookies. Vitamins C and K are also thought to ease symptoms; these can be found in fresh blackcurrants, kiwi fruit, peppers, and spinach. A lack of vitamin B6 has been linked with pregnancy nausea, so eat whole grains, potatoes, milk, cod, and bananas, which are all good sources.

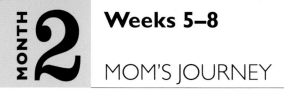
Going out/staying in

You probably haven't told many people you are pregnant yet, which can make work and social situations tricky. How do you handle fatigue, nausea, and not drinking without giving the secret away?

✳ Make a few changes

Your body is working overtime and you aren't alone if you feel tired at work or on your commute. Many women choose not to make their pregnancy common knowledge at work until the first trimester is safely over, but talking to a sympathetic boss or human resources manager could help make this stage of pregnancy easier. A boss who's in on your secret will be more understanding if your productivity flags, and it won't look suspicious when you take a long lunch for a prenatal doctor appointment. You may be able to negotiate flexible hours to avoid rush hour, and working from home occasionally can be a huge help if you're suffering from morning sickness.

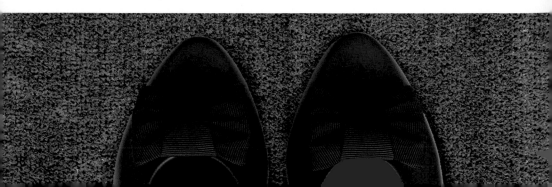

✳ Eating out

Your tastes can change in the early weeks of pregnancy, so you may not want your usual favorites. Since you need to eat regularly, late dinners might not work for you. Snack beforehand if you have to, but perhaps make plans for lunch instead of dinner.

✳ Alcohol-free

If you're known as someone who enjoys a drink in social situations, declining a glass can make heads turn. To keep the secret for a while longer, volunteer to drive when out with friends. You could choose drinks that look similar, such as grape juice instead of red wine.

✳ Change your routine

Why not plan to meet at the movie theater rather than a crowded bar; you will be guaranteed a seat! Or invite people to your home, where you can lounge with your feet up and serve just the food and beverages you like (or even order it in). But maybe the best nights, for a while, will be the ones you spend on the sofa with a good DVD wearing your pajamas. Relaxation is the new hedonism.

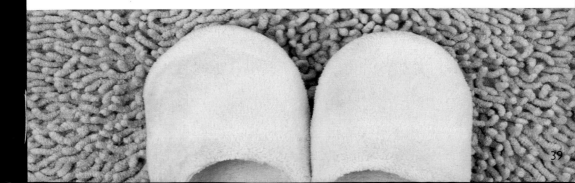

This month, the head makes up roughly half the length of your baby.

Budding and unfurling

By now you can just make out the form of your rapidly developing baby—rounded inward in a C-shape. Even at this early stage, many key body parts are taking shape and maneuvering into position.

✳ The little gray cells

By week five, a dark line of cells emerges along the back of the embryo, reflecting the final position of the spinal cord. At the top are two "lobes" that fold and develop into the neural tube. These changes are the start of the central nervous system, including the spinal cord and brain. From around six weeks, brain activity can be detected.

✳ A beating heart

The heart develops this month as no more than a tube, but it is in its final position at the front of the embryo. It begins beating around 21 days after conception and this can be picked up on an ultrasound, though you won't be able to hear it on a Doppler device (heart detector) for a while yet. Shortly afterward, it will flex into an S-shape so that the parts that will become the organ and atria are

Baby's progress bar: you are now 20% complete

LOADING ...

| 10% | 20% | 30% | 40% | 50% |

DID YOU KNOW?

BABY RESEMBLES a tadpole in shape—at six weeks she has a tail, but this soon deteriorates and by eight weeks has practically gone.

HOW BIG?
Your baby is now the size of a blackberry.

in the correct place. From here, four chambers separate. A precursor to blood starts to circulate through key blood vessels—at this point made up almost entirely of red blood cells.

✳ Early tummy

Another tube makes itself visible from week five—this one extending all the way from your baby's mouth to her tail end, and will eventually become her entire digestive system. All the organs she'll need to process and expel food emerge from this one simple tube.

✳ Budding limbs

Tiny bumps swell at the sides of the embryo from around weeks six and seven, which mark the beginnings of limbs. The arms and legs will lengthen out from these buds, like paddles or flippers, with ridges at the ends that transform into hands and feet. Soon there will be discernible fingers and toes, and by the end of the month the webbing that connects them will have all but vanished.

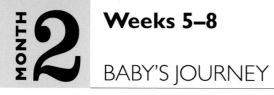

Take 400 mcg of folic acid daily to safeguard development of your baby's neural tube.

Baby's first face

At the beginning of month two, your baby's head is large in proportion to the rest of his body, but by week eight you'll be able to make out a distinctly human-shaped face.

✳ Big head

By week six your baby has gill-like features at the top of his body, which will evolve over the next few weeks into a face. Inside a large head, his brain is developing five distinct sections and nerve cells are connecting up the wiring that will link your baby's brain with every other part of his body via neural pathways. By the end of this month, his neck has started to stretch out from his head, which becomes more rounded and recognizably human in shape.

42

YOUR BABY IS officially a fetus from eight weeks onward. This stems from the Latin word for "young one" or "offspring."

150
The number of beats per minute of the fetal heart by week six.

❋ Face building

Bones are starting to replace cartilage and fuse together in the face, and as tissue joins together, recognizable features including the nose, forehead, cheeks, upper lip, and jaw become visible. Teeth buds are beginning to grow inside the jaw, and a rudimentary tongue is evident in his emerging palate. Openings appear for the nostrils, too.

❋ Fresh eyes

A large, dark circle at each side of your baby's face indicates that his eyes are now developing. Pigment is already detectable in the early retina, and, by week eight, the optic nerves connecting each eye to the brain have developed, and eyelids have grown over his eyes.

❋ Early ears

The internal structures of the ears start to form around week six, also forging connections to the developing brain. The external parts of the ear form as dips on the surface of the head, spaced wide apart on either side.

❋ Skin layering

At the beginning of week five your baby's skin is composed of one simple layer, but two weeks later it has developed a top layer, known as the "periderm," and a basal (base) layer. Tiny hair follicles also start to form in the skin at about this stage, but you won't find any actual hair growing until next month.

Being tired is your body's way of telling you to ease up—stress during pregnancy can raise your blood pressure, so take it easy. Luckily, this early fatigue will improve in the second trimester.

Relax and take it easy

You are pregnant, but the phone still rings, the laundry still piles up, and work deadlines loom as large as life. The key to managing stress when you are pregnant is to take care of yourself.

✳ Stress less

It's been proven that for most people a healthy diet, combined with plenty of sleep and relaxation, reduces stress and generally makes life easier. And these things are even more important now that your body is working hard to make a baby. Take a step back, and stay on top. By taking care of yourself you are taking care of your baby, too.

Eating well

- Eat breakfast daily
- Eat frequent, small meals
- Keep hydrated (see page 108)
- Make nutritious snacks
- Eat plenty of fruit and vegetables
- Cut out alcohol and caffeine

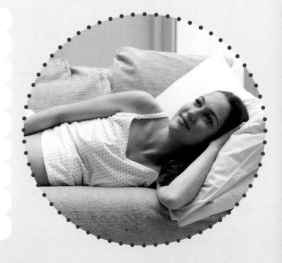

EXERCISE is one of the best stress-busters since it triggers the release of mood-enhancing endorphins—see pages 210–215 for easy, helpful pregnancy exercises.

ASK YOUR PARTNER FOR A BACK MASSAGE OR FOOT RUBS.

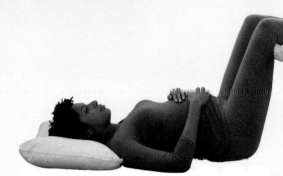

❋ Slow down

Find a window in each day to take a deep breath, relax, and do something for yourself. Look at the tips in the box, left, for a selection of ideas.

Ways to relax

- Join a pregnancy yoga or Pilates class
- Go for a walk
- Listen to music
- Lie down for a 15 minute power nap
- Take a daily lunch break when at work
- Enjoy a trip to the movies
- Indulge in a professional pregnancy massage
- Read a book or magazine
- Have a good chat with a friend
- Take a soothing shower or bath
- Go swimming
- Try a relaxing therapy (see page 104)
- Watch a funny movie or TV show

❋ Travel advice

You don't need to stop traveling just because you are pregnant, although it's a good idea to reduce the hassle if you can, and excessive travel should be avoided if possible. When traveling on a long-haul flight, help yourself by moving around the cabin, eating nutritious snacks, and drinking plenty of fluids. If commuting by train or bus, feel free to ask for a seat, and if the rush hour is particularly difficult, think about asking your boss if you can start and end your working day later to avoid it.

How do you do that?
AMAZING FACTS:
PREGNANT BODY

1 ### Expanding
In just 40 weeks, the uterus expands from the size of a pear to a size similar to that of a small watermelon. It increases in weight from 2½ oz (70 g) to around 2 lb 4 oz (1 kg).

2 ### Creating
During pregnancy, a woman creates a whole new organ—the placenta. This is the only organ that you get rid of after use! It works hard to deliver oxygen and nutrients to the baby.

3 ### Pumping
A pregnant woman has 50 percent more blood than usual by 20 weeks, and her cardiac output (volume pumped by each heartbeat) is 40 percent higher. She will also manufacture 20 percent more red blood cells to carry oxygen around her body.

4 ### Growing
The heart and liver may grow to meet the considerable demands of their extra workload; they will then return to their usual size after the birth.

5 ### Stretching
The hormone relaxin reduces cartilage and ligament density throughout the body so that the pelvis will be flexible for delivery. It also allows the rib cage to expand and accommodate an increased lung capacity.

BEING ABLE TO GROW A NEW PERSON in just 40 weeks is pretty amazing. There is a whole range of changes going on in your body to help you perform this incredible feat.

Glowing

The fabled pregnancy glow is real—a combination of enlarged blood vessels, increased blood volume, and more active oil glands causes a softer, rosier complexion.

Detcoting

Expectant mothers have a heightened sense of smell, thought to have evolved to help detect the small amounts of toxins in food and liquids that could be dangerous to an unborn baby. It can make you dislike the smell of cigarettes, coffee, and alcohol.

Consuming

An extra 200 calories a day is sufficient for a pregnant woman to nourish her baby, who takes whatever nutrients he needs first, leaving her with the leftovers. In order to ensure maximum absorption of nutrients, digestion slows down during this time.

Beautifying

An expectant mom's hair gets thicker and glossier due to the estrogen receptors it contains, and the fact that hair loss is reduced. It will also grow quicker, as will fingernails and toenails.

Protecting

By 39 weeks the uterus will contain around 35 fl oz (1 liter) of amniotic fluid. At 99.5°F (37.5°C), this protective bubble of fluid is warmer than your body temperature, and is a little like saltwater. It is replaced gradually, every three hours during pregnancy.

Weeks 5–8
DAD'S SURVIVAL
GUIDE

DID YOU KNOW?

Raging hormones

Pregnancy hormones are kicking in, so your partner might experience "morning sickness" (a misnomer since it can occur any time), fatigue, mood changes, and nausea, or she may be lucky and sail through it all.

✳ Swings and merry-go-rounds

A cocktail of pregnancy hormones is flooding your partner, and she may start to feel the side effects. She may feel irritable one moment and elated the next, full of energy and enthusiasm at lunchtime and exhausted after work. This is due to a chemical reaction in the brain that affects the mood-regulating neurotransmitters, which in turn can destabilize her mood. Combine that with any anxiety about the coming months, and it can be a pretty tiring time for you both. Talking about your partner's concerns can help her to cope, and keep in mind that it probably isn't you she's getting angry with.

✳ Dawning sickness

The same hormones that cause mood swings can also make some women feel very sick, known as morning sickness. This affects people differently—some women may vomit, while others have an intense sensation of nausea akin to motion or seasickness. It can occur in the morning, or be stronger when tired at the end of the day, or during the night. Some expectant moms feel terrible

SOMETIMES dads can develop Couvade syndrome (phantom pregnancy).

MOST WOMEN suffer from nausea at some point, but the good news is that it usually subsides by the fourth month of pregnancy.

BRING YOUR PARTNER A GINGER COOKIE IN BED TO HELP WITH NAUSEA.

IF YOUR PARTNER has lost her appetite, cook something delicious containing ginger to help alleviate nausea. A stir-fry would be great.

around the clock. If your partner feels nauseous you need to be aware of just how debilitating it can be to feel so ill—imagine a crippling hangover! Nausea can make it hard to continue with everyday life, such as traveling, cooking, and eating your usual meals. It can also bring an awareness that her body is no longer her own, and that lack of control can be pretty scary.

✳ Your growing baby

By the end of month two, your baby is now a "fetus" and has tiny arm and leg buds and facial features. His central nervous system and heart are developing. He is starting to move, but you and your partner won't be able to feel this yet since there is plenty of space in there!

Do

Encourage your partner to rest, and help with shared jobs as much as possible. Get some early nights.

———————————

Go out and enjoy yourselves when you both feel like it.

———————————

Take a walk together for some fresh air and exercise.

Don't

Eat or cook strong-smelling foods, since this may trigger her nausea.

———————————

Call the doctor every time your partner is sick. But if she can't keep food or liquid down, then make an appointment.

———————————

Smoke near your partner—this may be absorbed by your growing baby. Try to quit!

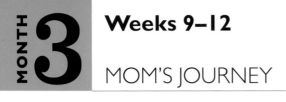

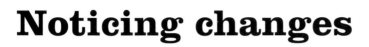

Noticing changes

There's no pretending now—this month you'll see a difference in your body as your breasts grow, your skin starts to change, and your waist thickens. Your anatomy ultrasound should help make everything seem more real.

✳ Need some support?

Your breasts have probably been the first part of your body to look and feel different: full, supersensitive, and definitely larger. You might find a sports bra more comfortable than your regular bra now. Even this early in pregnancy your body is preparing your breasts to feed your baby. Until now this has been caused by increased levels of estrogen and progesterone, but there's a new hormone in the mix—**human placental lactogen** (HPL), produced by the placenta. This increases the amount of sugar in your blood in order to transfer nutrients to your baby. It also prepares the mammary glands for making milk. You'll probably have noticed the areola (the area around your nipples) becoming larger and darker. Can you spot any new little white bumps there? Known as **Montgomery's tubercles**, these enlarged sebaceous glands produce a protective antibacterial oil that keeps the skin clean and smooth.

✳ Feeling dizzy?

The blood vessels in your body have been relaxing and getting wider (dilating) over the last few weeks, thanks to your increased hormones, particularly progesterone. This dilation allows your veins to hold more

23%

MORE BLOOD is pumped to your uterus by week 12 than before you were pregnant.

GOOD TO EAT
Eggs for B vitamins and choline, and to boost folic acid absorption.

blood, ensuring all the new blood vessels in the placenta have a plentiful supply and that those organs that are working harder, such as your kidneys, are well supported. Your body is manufacturing more plasma and red blood cells this month, but neither are up to capacity, meaning your blood pressure is likely to be lower than usual. So if you stand up quickly you may feel dizzy. Try to bring your head up last in order to give the blood time to reach your brain. Faintness may also result from dipping blood-sugar levels; snacking on carbohydrates can help, and don't skip meals.

NEW WORDS
- HPL
- Montgomery's tubercles
- Spider nevi

✱ Is it hot in here?

Have you noticed you feel warmer, particularly your hands and feet? Are there tiny new veins on the surface of your skin, especially on your breasts and legs? The two changes are connected: more blood is flowing to your skin through the veins (called **spider nevi**) to release the excess heat generated by your increased metabolism and blood flow.

✱ Where's the bathroom?

Though you might not notice a huge difference in your figure yet, your uterus has started to enlarge and thicken. It's likely to be pressing on your bladder, which can make you want to urinate at unexpected moments. You may find you're having to get up at night, too—your kidneys are working harder to filter the extra blood circulating, which means more urine. Unfortunately, this is an aspect of pregnancy that, as your baby and your uterus enlarge, will only get worse!

Your pelvic muscles start stretching from now on, so start Kegel exercises.

Fact or fiction?

You may be getting plenty of (un)welcome advice at the moment about the most ordinary things. Is it really dangerous to eat cheese, or paint the baby's room? Does your cat have to move out? What are the facts?

✳ Weighing the risks

Parenthood is about assessing risk: getting acquainted with facts and opinions, working out what you and your partner think about them, and trusting your judgment enough to put those thoughts into action. Often you are just going to have to do your best.

✳ Getting tipsy before the test

Did you have a few drinks too many before you knew you were pregnant? Studies in the media sometimes suggest this might be risky for your baby, so if you are really concerned talk to your doctor. However, try not to worry since most women find everything is fine. Instead, channel any anxiety into positive change, such as quitting for now.

✳ Dubious decorating

There's convincing evidence to stop you from renovating rooms that haven't been touched since the 1970s since the paint is likely to contain lead, and sanding or stripping it releases this heavy metal into the air. Exposure may harm your baby's developing brain and nervous and reproductive systems. Choose paints, thinners, varnishes, and sealants

DID YOU KNOW?

INCREASING YOUR VITAMIN C intake will strengthen your veins and may help to prevent spider veins.

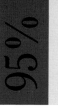

95%

OF WOMEN felt more reassured after an ultrasound in their first trimester.

with low volatile organic compound (VOC) content, which is clearly marked on the container. And if you are concerned, it's a great excuse to put your feet up and have someone else do the work—using eco-friendly materials, of course.

✳ Sex in pregnancy

You might have the idea that sex during pregnancy could be harmful for your baby. Actually, sex is something you can enjoy throughout pregnancy, unless your doctor says otherwise. Thanks to your hormones you may feel like more of it than ever before!

✳ Household chemicals

A 2013 report by the Royal College of Obstetricians and Gynecologists warned pregnant women to avoid chemicals in cleaning products, cosmetics, and common plastics. The US Department of Health and Human Services also recommends that pregnant women steer clear of a variety of household chemicals, including cleaning products, paint, and pest-control products which contain volatile organic compounds that can lead to indoor air pollution. This is because the chlorine, ammonia, solvents, and pesticides that necessitate these cautions can trigger nausea, irritate your skin, and respiratory tract, or affect the central nervous system.

✳ Furry creatures

There is no reason to ask your cat, dog, or chickens to move out, but you do need to be superconscious about hygiene now you are pregnant. Avoid dealing with cat litter or poop of any kind, and wear gloves for any mucky jobs. Avoid flea treatments and get advice from your vet about natural options.

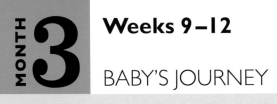

MONTH 3

Weeks 9–12

BABY'S JOURNEY

Your baby is already a boy or a girl although you won't be able to tell on an ultrasound for a few weeks yet.

All in place

A tiny person is starting to emerge from the cells. Your baby's organs are already grown and are starting to work, and she has an enormous head!

✳ Over the first hurdle

By the end of week 12 your baby will have completed the first and most vital stage of the journey, when critical development takes place in every body system and all the basics of human physiology are put in place. Your baby now looks like an actual tiny person!

✳ Heart-to-heart

By week 10, your baby's heart has developed into the definitive four-chambered heart. The two atria receive blood from the fetal circulation, while the ventricles pump blood out to the lungs and the rest of your baby's body. Valves develop at the exit of all four chambers to ensure that the blood is always pumped in one direction.

✳ Stretching out

By now your baby's torso looks straighter. The arms and legs are fully formed with visible elbows, wrists, and ankles that can move, and the

Baby's progress bar: you are now 30% complete

LOADING ...

| 10% | 20% | 30% | 40% | 50% |

DID YOU
KNOW?

BY WEEK 12 your baby weighs
$^1/_2$–1 oz (15–30 g). Moving around
inside you helps her develop a
strong skeleton and muscles.

HOW BIG?
She is roughly the
size of a plum.

limbs are lengthening. After week 10, tiny fingernails and toenails will appear and webbing between the fingers and toes will disappear.

❋ Muscle action

The first movements a fetus makes are small involuntary twitches, since the nervous system is not yet developed enough for the brain and body parts to talk to each other. Movement starts to increase in frequency in the third month, though you won't be able feel it for another month or so.

❋ Home sweet home

Your baby continues to float freely within amniotic fluid, which cushions her from knocks and bumps. The amniotic sac is surrounded by an inner and outer layer, which are separated by a space that contains the yolk sac.

❋ Future generations

Externally, the genitals are well developed by week 12, while inside the fetus, cells are growing that will eventually form sperm or eggs.

Mouth can open and close.

Heart rate is about 160 beats per minute.

Ears are nearly in their final position on the head.

The placenta

By the end of this month, the placenta is fully developed, ready to support your baby until birth by delivering nutrients and oxygen, taking away waste products, and providing protection.

✳ Layering and connecting

The placenta began its development in month one, just after implantation, when layers of chorion and amnion membrane were forming on the wall of your uterus around the embryo. Those layers have now thickened and extended to form a flat, oval sac filled with amniotic fluid, usually attached to the top or side of your uterus. By week 10 you have about 1 fl oz (30 ml) of amniotic fluid (mostly water). This increases little by little until you eventually have around 35 fl oz (1 liter) toward the end of the third trimester.

✳ Life-support system

The main role of the placenta is to supply your baby with oxygen and nutrients and to take away waste. Within the chorion membrane are 200 villi, containing blood vessels, grouped like bunches of grapes. Longer villi reach deep into the wall of your uterus to bring in oxygenated blood from your arteries. These have widened and are delivering more blood to your uterus than before pregnancy, thanks to the extra blood circulating and your increased heart rate. Your blood pools in the placenta. Here the bunches of smaller villi bathe

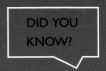

DID YOU
KNOW?

SOME COMPANIES OFFER the opportunity to pay to store stem cells from your baby's umbilical cord to treat future diseases.

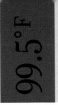

99.5°F

At 99.5°F (37.5°C), amniotic fluid is warmer than your body temperature.

in it and absorb oxygen and nutrients via their tips where the layer of cells is very thin. At the same time, waste products, including carbon dioxide, transfer to your veins and are carried away to your lungs and kidneys to be processed and expelled.

✳ Umbilical cord

Your baby is connected to the placenta by an umbilical cord, which starts at his navel and is also now fully developed. Within the cord is a main vein, transferring fresh blood filled with oxygen and nutrients into your baby's bloodstream. It also houses two arteries that carry used blood, containing carbon dioxide and other waste, away out to your body. These three vessels wind around each other to create a coil covered in sticky jelly and a layer of membrane.

✳ Protective shield

Amniotic fluid provides a cushioning, temperature-controlled environment for your baby, while the surrounding membranes create a barrier from harmful substances, from bacteria to environmental toxins. Later in pregnancy, the placenta passes on antibodies to protect your newborn. However, the placenta cannot protect against viruses, such as rubella, listeria bacteria (found in soil and some soft cheeses), or heavy metals, such as lead, that may enter the bloodstream.

✳ Hormone factory

From now on, the placenta is responsible for manufacturing the hCG, estrogen, and progesterone required until the end of pregnancy to prepare your body for childbirth and breast feeding.

MONTH 3

You can now have 3D sonograms and video recordings of the first ultrasound, which can often be taken home with you.

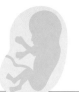

You will find out your estimated date of delivery (EDD).

The first ultrasound

Around 12 weeks you may be given your first ultrasound. This sonogram image enables you and medical staff to see your baby for the first time.

✻ What's it for?

This ultrasound helps your medical team calculate your baby's exact age and estimate when he might be born— his EDD (Estimated Date of Delivery). This preliminary ultrasound also helps check other things, such as how many babies you are carrying (one or more!), and your baby's heartbeat. Although the ultrasound is not specifically for picking up abnormalities, sometimes problems can be detected.

NUCHAL TRANSLUCENCY SCAN

This ultrasound may be given during 11–14 weeks of pregnancy to screen for Down syndrome and other conditions. It measures the thickness of the pocket of fluid (the nuchal fold) behind your baby's neck and, combined with a simple blood test, can be used to calculate risk.

✻ How do I prepare?

You might be asked to have a full bladder, because this helps push your uterus up for a clear image. Be aware that occasionally ultrasounds can show unexpected things, but otherwise, just look forward to it!

✻ What happens?

A sonographer will do your ultrasound. You will be asked to lie down and pull your top up, and possibly your pants or skirt down a little to expose your abdomen. The sonographer will smooth a gel over your belly and then

TOP TIP

LOOK FOR THE LETTERS CRL on your sonogram. This is your baby's "crown-to-rump length." This figure gives an accurate estimate of age.

5% **OF BABIES ARE** delivered on their predicted due date.

press down with a handheld device linked to a computer screen. He or she may move the device around to get a clearer image of your baby.

✳ Will it hurt?

It shouldn't hurt, though the gel rubbed over your belly might feel cold and the probe might prod a little; at worst it may just feel a little uncomfortable. The baby won't be able to feel anything!

✳ Who can I take?

Usually you can bring one adult along with you. You may want to bring the baby's father, your mom, or a close friend. Children are sometimes not permitted, depending on your health-care provider.

✳ How do they do it?

The device sends high frequency sound waves, inaudible to the human ear, into your abdomen and records the echoes which bounce back with a tiny microphone. A 2D-image is built up from the echoes.

Your sonogram

You may feel that you are supposed to know just what is what in your baby's first image, but if you find the blobby white and dark patches of your sonogram baffling, rest assured you would not be the first parent to feel this. Solid structures, such as bone and muscle, appear as white or gray, while soft tissues, such as the eyeballs or empty structures, including the heart's chambers, will appear dark red or black.

This baby's profile is very clear. You can see the nose, mouth, and eyes as he moves around.

The eye sockets appear as dark hollows in the clear profile of the skull. Eyes are soft tissue so appear dark.

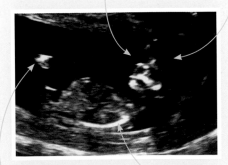

Is that a foot or a hand? Solid white areas show bone, and if the areas are moving, it is likely to be a foot or hand.

The spine is clearly visible as a solid, white, curved line.

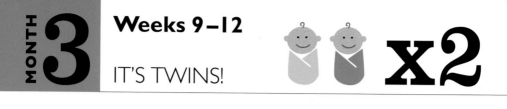

Expecting more than one?

You've just gotten used to the idea of being pregnant, when you discover that it's not just one! Wow! It's perfectly natural to feel overwhelmed as well as excited; there is a lot to take in.

✴ Tip-top care

Your pregnancy will most likely go smoothly with few, if any, complications, but you will be given extra prenatal appointments to help ensure that all is well. The chance of you developing high blood pressure, preeclampsia, and diabetes is raised, and so you will be monitored for these conditions. Extra ultrasounds will check that your babies are growing at a similar rate. This is especially relevant when identical twins share a placenta because more blood may circulate to one baby (twin-to-twin transfusion syndrome).

✴ How are you feeling?

High levels of the pregnancy hormone hCG can lead to you experiencing nausea, sickness, and fatigue, and it is usually worse when carrying more than one baby. The good news is that this should improve after the first trimester. Two or more babies means there is less room in your body, which can lead to heartburn and indigestion as your uterus presses against other organs. Eating small

Try to eat six small meals each day—this will help to alleviate any indigestion. Eat a nutrient-rich diet to support your body, and include good sources of fiber, since carrying twins and triplets can increase constipation due to the pressure on your bowel.

and regular meals can alleviate this. There's also a greater risk of developing anemia than with one baby, so eat plenty of iron-rich foods. If you experience back and pelvic pain, seek help from your doctor—supportive clothing and correcting your posture may help.

✳ Room for two

Your belly will probably expand sooner, and by as early as 10 weeks it can be hard to conceal a belly! You will almost certainly gain more weight than with one baby due to the extra amniotic fluid and larger placenta/s, but the figures may not be as dramatic as you expect. Women carrying one baby gain around 24lb (11kg); an extra baby usually means a weight gain of just an extra 10lb (4.5kg) or so.

✳ Planning the delivery

Your delivery is likely to be at, or before, 37 weeks, so you need to plan to leave work earlier, get your hospital bag packed, have two car seats installed, and have baby clothes chosen. 37 weeks is considered full term for a twins pregnancy; the placenta/s have worked hard and you are probably ready to deliver! While a cesarean is likely, there's no reason not to plan for a natural delivery as long as your babies are in a good position, with the first twin head down (cephalic position).

IVF TWIN RATES
The rise in IVF treatments has increased twin rates dramatically. Figures show that in recent years, 1 in 30 babies born in the US have been twins, compared to 1 in 53 babies in 1980.

There is regular debate about the ideal age at which to have a baby. After 35 years of age the number and quality of your eggs is reduced. But then again, it takes only one to make a baby!

Older moms

Many women now have babies later in life—nearly 40% of American women who waited until 35–44 have had at least two children. Is it really something to worry about and what are the real risks and benefits?

✳ A solid start

Studies of older moms highlight many convincing arguments for delaying motherhood. Becoming a mom slightly later in life means you are more likely to be in a settled, stable relationship, be better educated, and be more financially secure. You're also more likely to have achieved goals in your professional life and to have reached a satisfactory status, making it easier to put your career on hold, and easier to return to it after the baby is born. Motherhood is likely to be something you embrace wholeheartedly since you're ready to focus on family, and you are less likely to feel tied down or fear you are missing out on other aspects of life. And long-term, you're more likely to achieve a fulfilling work-life balance.

✳ Confident parenting

Accruing life experience before embarking on motherhood increases self-confidence, and older moms are likely to have the necessary life skills and perspective to cope well with the ups and downs of

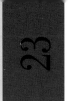

DID YOU KNOW?

WOMEN WHO GIVE BIRTH when over 40 years old are four times as likely to live to be 100 than younger moms.

23

THE MEAN AGE OF WOMEN IN THE US HAVING THEIR FIRST BABY.

parenting, as well as having a clear parenting style in mind. One study found that children of older mothers tend to do well academically.

✳ What about the health risks?

If you are 35 years or older and expecting your first baby, you are termed "elderly primigravida"; you will be monitored closely during your pregnancy and offered extra checks for genetic abnormalities. Women in this age bracket are more likely to develop conditions such as high blood pressure and diabetes, and run a higher risk of having a low-lying placenta. During labor, medical interventions and cesareans are also more common. Try to see this extra level of care as a bonus; you and your baby are in safe hands. And remember, the majority of older women have healthy pregnancies and babies. Also, since older moms are likely to have a good fitness regimen, eat healthily, and be less likely to smoke than younger women, this will help you to deal with any extra fatigue you may feel when baby arrives!

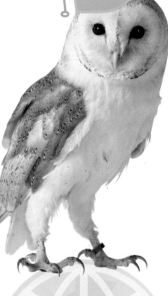

IN THE US, the birth rate has fallen in recent years, while the average age of first-time moms has risen to 23 years.

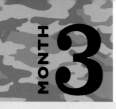

Weeks 9–12
DAD'S SURVIVAL
GUIDE

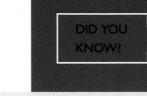

The secret's out

It's nearly time for the dating scan. Once you have confirmation that all is well, you can start shouting the news from the rooftops and it will all seem more real.

✳ Say cheese

The 11–14-week scan will be the first of many images of your baby. The purpose of this scan is to check that this is a viable fetus that is developing normally. The good news is that in most cases all is well and once you have heard the heartbeat for the first time the risk of miscarriage drops to just five percent. Scans are not harmful to your partner or baby; they can be slightly uncomfortable though since she will need a really full bladder for the scan to work effectively. The sonographer will take measurements to predict the due date more accurately; he or she will also check whether there is just one baby (or maybe more!), and look for any abnormalities in the development of spine, limbs, and organs.

✳ Start spreading the news

If you've been keeping the pregnancy secret until this point, now is the time to start broadcasting your happy news. Do you tell the grandparents, siblings, or close friends first? Perhaps wait until all the key

YOUR PARTNER MAY START to get heartburn and indigestion as pregnancy hormones have relaxed the valve at the top of her stomach, allowing acid to escape.

YOUR BABY HAS JUST DEVELOPED REFLEXES AND MAY RESPOND TO GENTLE TOUCH.

Do

Move mountains to get to the scan. It's a once-in-a-lifetime experience that you should see.

Ask questions if you want to. It can be quite hard to tell what is what on the scan.

Keep the picture. People will love to see it, and it's a great souvenir!

Don't

Panic at the scan. Chances are that everything will be just fine.

Worry if people are shocked by your news. Your happiness is what matters.

Forget to tell all your key players first. You need to keep them in your corner since they'll be crucial support in the months and years ahead.

players in your life have heard it directly from you before you announce it on the internet. Don't worry if everyone's reaction isn't what you thought it would be; you might have friends who tell you it's hard work, you'll never sleep again, and some might be jealous. Everyone has a different life plan, so try not to take it personally.

✳ Talking it out

Now that the news is out, you may find you are on the receiving end of advice. There is so much information out there (the internet is a mixed blessing) that it can be great to allay concerns by canvassing opinion from people you trust. Experienced dads can be great sounding boards, and talking to someone who knows what you're going through can be reassuring. Later you might meet other parents at childbirth classes—you obviously have at least one thing in common.

WHAT ARE YOUR PLANS when baby arrives? Who's going to take care of him and for how long? Maybe you'd like to?

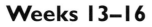

Starting to bloom

Welcome to the second trimester of pregnancy! The most disorienting part of the journey is over, and any nausea should start to lift now. Most exciting of all, you will start to develop a visible belly.

✳ Looking pregnant at last

Depending on your body shape and the strength of your core muscles, you should start to develop a tiny belly by week 16. Your doctor can now feel the uterus in your abdomen. Though your breasts will stop feeling so tender, they too are developing— by the end of this month the milk-producing glands will be fully primed to manufacture breast milk.

✳ What's going on inside?

Your red-blood-cell count is increasing rapidly to carry the extra oxygen your body needs to feed the placenta and baby. You also have additional plasma to deal with the increased blood flow to your organs, skin, and kidneys. Your heart is working twice as hard, while your digestive system is slowing down.

✳ Health complaints

Symptoms including a stuffy nose, blocked ears, swollen, bleeding gums, and snoring are all common at this stage of pregnancy. Feel reassured, they are a sign that your body is doing just what it needs

DID YOU KNOW?

YOUR BLOOD volume starts to increase now, causing a noticeable pregnancy "glow."

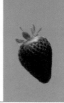

GOOD TO EAT
Strawberries and blueberries since their vitamin C content aids iron absorption.

to keep you and your baby healthy. Increased circulation sends more blood through your mucous membranes, which causes slight swelling in all the tissue lining parts of your body that are in contact with the air, such as your nose, windpipe, and lungs.

✳ Help, I'm changing color!

It's quite normal for your nipples and genitals to get darker because you now have more pigment-bearing cells. You might notice a fine line developing down your tummy from your navel to your pubic bone—this is called the linea nigra. You may also develop darker or uneven patches of skin on your cheekbones, forehead, nose, and chin, called melasma or chloasma (years ago it was called the "mask of pregnancy"). All skin pigmentation changes usually fade once the baby is born, so don't worry too much. They do, however, increase and get darker with exposure to sun, so use a high-SPF sunscreen to help minimize any long-term changes. Your skin is more sensitive, too, so you need extra protection against burning and long-term damage.

STRETCH MARK ALERT

Up to 80 percent of pregnant women notice reddish-brown streaks, called **striae gravidarum**, caused when the body grows rapidly. These spiderlike lines fade to silver, but to keep skin stretchy and to reduce the amount of lines or any itching, gently massage your belly, breasts, hips, and thighs with a rich body lotion. Olive oil is used for this purpose worldwide.

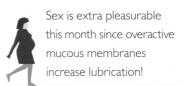

Sex is extra pleasurable this month since overactive mucous membranes increase lubrication!

Spreading the news

As your energy returns this month and mood swings calm down, you're likely to feel less anxious and more able to relax into your pregnancy. You might be ready to tell friends and colleagues at work.

✳ Relax and settle in

Your hormones are starting to calm down and the risk of miscarriage is far lower than in the first trimester, so this tends to be when people start spreading the news. You're likely to feel more positive and energetic, and you can channel this into practical matters, such as researching options for birth, or planning childbirth classes.

✳ When to tell

It's tempting to shout the good news to friends, family, and colleagues right away, but once the news is out it can dominate conversation and social

DID YOU KNOW?

YOU ARE LESS LIKELY to need to urinate so often now since your uterus has grown and moved out of the pelvic cavity.

45%

BY THIS MONTH'S END, YOUR BODY WILL CONTAIN 45% MORE BLOOD.

events, so make sure you are ready. If your belly is not showing yet, you may want to keep quiet at work while you find out more about employment rights. Pregnancy can affect workplace politics since colleagues may start to reassess your capabilities or maneuver into position for when your maternity leave begins.

> *Your breasts are already making colostrum—baby's first milk.*

✳ Treat yourself

Mark this new stage of your pregnancy journey by buying clothes that flaunt and flatter your changing shape. Low-cut jeans, long tops, and stretchy wrap dresses can work just as well as maternity wear, especially in the early months. You'll need maternity clothes by the third trimester and post-delivery, too, and will get heartily sick of them, so adapt your regular clothes for as long as possible.

✳ Dealing with the attention

Once you tell all, you'll find you become public property. Being the focus of good wishes, gifts, and smiles can be delightful, and it can be a great way to meet new people and talk to colleagues you've never met before. But everyone has a birth horror story or tales of sleepless nights to share, and some may want to hug or pat your belly. Prepare some polite but firm responses to preserve your privacy, just in case!

A tiny person

Your baby has completed perhaps the most tricky part of the pregnancy journey. By week 13, all the major organs and body systems have developed, and her muscles are growing stronger.

✳ Communication system

Nerves to and from your baby's brain are being coated in a protective layer of fat, called myelin, which will allow messages to travel between the brain and muscles in the rest of the body.

✳ Getting active

Muscles are able to contract and relax now, so your baby can move, stretching out her limbs, turning around inside you, and clasping both hands together. This can be detected on an ultrasound, so you can enjoy watching the movements at your 12-week scan. If you press your belly, your baby will respond by wiggling, though you can't feel it yet because of the amniotic fluid that cushions her.

Baby's progress bar: you are now 40% complete

LOADING ...

10%　　　20%　　　30%　　　40%　　　50%

BY 16 WEEKS your baby weighs about 3¼ oz (90 g) and is 4–5 in (10–12 cm) long. Your baby will grow 2 in (5 cm) this month.

HOW BIG? She is about the size of an orange.

✳ Drinking and urinating

The kidneys start to work this month, and your baby will swallow the amniotic fluid she is floating in. She starts to make urine, and passes it out into the amniotic sac.

✳ Independent living

By the end of this month your baby will be creating red blood cells inside her body —in the bone marrow, liver, and spleen— rather than depending on an outside source. Your baby and placenta are also now producing hormones themselves (taking over from your ovary), including estrogen and all the progesterone required until birth.

✳ Boy or girl?

Your baby is now visibly a boy or a girl, since the "differentiation" process is complete by week 14. Ovarian follicles, or a prostate gland, have started to appear and the external sex organs are evident, although they are too small to see on a sonogram.

Brain is developing to send messages to the rest of the body.

Placenta measures about ½ in (1 cm) thick and about 3 in (8 cm) across.

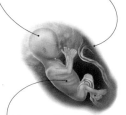

Heart and lungs are now formed.

60%   70%   80%   90%   100%

Your baby is now growing a neck, which makes his head look more upright.

New sensory world

Your baby's eyes and ears develop rapidly this month and he will be able to hear and see. Taste buds and nerve endings develop, too, so he can feel things as he moves around. But it's probably too soon to taste.

"It's pretty noisy in here!"

✳ Sound

Your baby's ears are moving into position on the sides of the head and the tiny bones inside are hardening. Once this happens, your baby can hear you from the inside (your beating heart, whooshing blood, and rumbling tummy), and can also detect sounds from the outside world, including your voice. His own vocal folds, or cords, develop in week 13.

BONDING WITH YOUR BABY starts before birth. Tune into his patterns of movement—speak softly to him when he is quiet and sing lively songs when more alert.

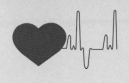

✳ Sight

Although your baby's eyelids remain closed, the eyes are fully formed—tiny eyelashes and eyebrows are even visible—and the retinas become sensitive to light. Your baby can see bright light coming in through your abdomen, which may start to help with distinguishing between night and day.

✳ Taste

Taste buds are emerging on his tongue, and 32 tooth buds are developing in the jawbones. Your baby is also practicing sucking in and swallowing amniotic fluid, but probably can't taste anything yet.

✳ Touch

Your developing baby can wiggle his toes and curl up his tiny fingers. His arms are long enough to make thumb-sucking possible.

✳ Expressions

The facial bones and muscles are all in place and your baby's face moves through a series of expressions—frowning, smirking, squinting, wrinkling the forehead, and pursing the lips—even though the brain isn't fully controlling any of the movements yet.

IN THE DEMOCRATIC REPUBLIC OF CONGO, mothers sing to their unborn babies, repeating a single song until the birth. After birth the mother will sing the same tune to comfort the child. It sounds like a great idea to try.

I forgot. Sorry!
COMMON COMPLAINTS IN MID-PREGNANCY

WHAT TO DO

1 Forgetfulness

You have suddenly turned into an airhead and keep forgetting things.

Write things down in a notepad or on your smartphone, or reduce the number of things you need to remember by delegating (though this is perhaps easier said than done!).

2 Clumsiness

You keep dropping your car keys, banging into things, and are generally clumsy.

Proceed with care. Slow down, use extra caution in the bath or shower, keep hallways and stairs clear, and don't even think about standing on any chairs to reach things.

3 Gas

You are bloated, gassy, and uncomfortable.

Reduce your intake of carbonated beverages, and sip warm water instead. Small, simple meals are best. Exercise helps, too, as does wearing loose clothing.

4 Heartburn

Acid reflux, a burning pain in your chest or stomach, feeling sick. Ugh!

Eight out of ten women get heartburn during pregnancy. Avoid triggers, such as orange juice, chocolate, spicy food, or peppermint tea. Eat little and often. Ask your doctor if you can take antacids.

5 Hair and nails

Your nails are more brittle, your hair has become curly, and you are growing a moustache.

You can safely pluck facial hair, but don't use bleaches and hair-removal creams. Wear rubber gloves for housework to protect your nails.

YOU SHOULD BE FEELING a lot better this trimester, and less tired. The extra estrogen you produce now may bring new symptoms.

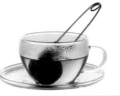

TOP TIP
Ask your doctor which herbal teas are safe to alleviate heartburn.

WHAT TO DO

6

Skin changes
You seem to be looking at a different face in the mirror. Is it really you?

Acne, spider veins, and pimply eruptions are all common in pregnancy. Use a cleanser to clear up pimples, and a high-SPF sunscreen to protect your skin when in the sun.

7

Pain in your groin
There are sharp stabbing pains in your groin and side.

This can be a sign of symphysis pubis dysfunction (see page 233) so tell your doctor about your symptoms. Be careful when getting in and out of the car or bath, and try not to do any heavy lifting.

8

Stuffy nose
You don't have a cold, but you feel blocked up and stuffy.

About 30 percent of pregnant women suffer from rhinitis during pregnancy. Try placing hot towels over the bridge of your nose or inhaling steam. Saline nose drops help, too.

9

Nosebleeds
If it's not a stuffy nose, it's a nosebleed!

Nosebleeds can happen much more frequently due to increased blood flow to the tissue lining your nose. To try to avoid nosebleeds, blow your nose gently, one nostril at a time.

10

Hot and sweaty
You wake up boiling hot, or suddenly feel hot and sweaty.

Wear layers of clothes—then you can shed them one by one if a hot flash hits you. Hot flashes will pass— at least until you hit menopause!

Top 10

75

4

TIME TO GO SHOPPING

BORROW items if you can; newborn clothes and toys rarely wear out.

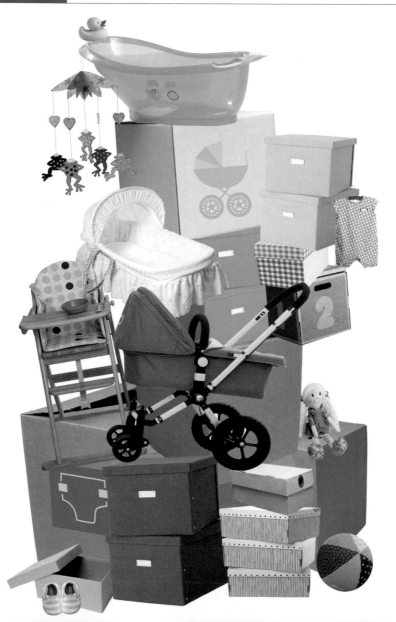

The bare essentials

You're getting ready for your great adventure into parenthood, but what will you need to get you through the first few months? In Finland, every new baby receives a cardboard box containing essential clothes and goods; the box then becomes a crib. That shows you how little you need. Here is our guide:

Basic gear (pages 92–3)
The equipment you will need in the first few weeks, from car seat and crib to baby monitors and a baby bath.

Hospital bag (pages 122–3)
You may be in the hospital for a while so make it as comfortable as you can.

Baby's wardrobe (pages 150–1)
Onesies, sleep suits, and a few hats. Newborns don't need a huge wardrobe, so save your money for the teenage years!

MONTH **4**

Weeks 13–16
DAD'S SURVIVAL
GUIDE

DID YOU
KNOW?

Getting busy

Right now you're heading into the second trimester. This part of the pregnancy should be easier for you and your partner since morning sickness should subside. She may get her energy back, and feel more like her usual self.

✳ Do a little dance

Both of you need to be in good shape for taking care of a small child. There is also evidence to suggest that your partner will have an easier labor and birth if she is fit. Three or four sessions of cardiovascular activity a week will do both of you a world of good, physically and emotionally (see page 210). If neither of you are athletic, get into the habit of taking brisk walks. You need to be careful with exercises where she might fall, or very intense exercise that raises her body temperature. That can all come when baby is older!

✳ Make a little love

There is one other great form of exercise you can do together—sex. Many women experience an increase in their usual sex drive during pregnancy due to hormonal changes. If your partner is one of the lucky ones, go ahead and enjoy the opportunity to bond. There are going to be a lot of changes once your baby arrives and your sex schedule may get somewhat disrupted by the ensuing sleepless nights.

EXPERIMENTS suggest women are more attracted to men who like babies.

BECAUSE YOUR PARTNER'S LIGAMENTS ARE MORE FLEXIBLE, SHE IS SUSCEPTIBLE TO INJURY. IF YOU EXERCISE TOGETHER, TAKE IT EASY.

YOUR BABY is now 5 in (12 cm) long and his rubbery skeleton is forming into real bones.

Some women feel the opposite, however, so give her time and find other ways to be close.

THE 20-WEEK ULTRASOUND is fast approaching. Are you going to find out the sex of your baby, or will you wait until the birth?

✱ Get down tonight

Many men wonder whether sex is safe in pregnancy and the simple answer is yes. Your baby is well protected in the amniotic sack as well as by the strong muscles of the uterus. You may find your libido is affected—maybe you find her swelling femininity highly erotic, or maybe you have started seeing her body as more functional than fun. Both of these are entirely normal; either way, you should celebrate the connection you share now that you have created a new life together.

Do

Go away for the weekend together, and make a fuss over your partner.

———————————

Enjoy sleeping in together—these mornings will soon be harder to come by.

———————————

Try out some new sex positions that are comfortable with the belly!

Don't

Worry if she doesn't feel like sex. Tell her how sexy her new curves are and she might change her mind.

———————————

Take your partner on a 10-mile jog or anything else too strenuous.

———————————

Forget that you need to be fit. There is a lot of running around to come in the future.

Halfway there

Week 20 is the halfway point in your journey and a cause to celebrate! You may feel baby flutter for the first time, which can be both weird and exciting. Your energy levels are high so enjoy it and get active.

✳ Tickled from the inside

The lovely word "quickening" is used to describe the sensation of feeling your baby's first movements. It can be tricky at first to recognize these fluttery, rolling sensations: is it your baby wiggling or is it gas? Quickening generally happens during weeks 20–25, but many second-time moms sense it sooner, from as early as week 13.

✳ Get moving

Make time for gentle exercise (see pages 210–215), especially if you felt too under the weather during your first trimester. Walking, swimming, yoga, and tai chi are all suitable. Pregnancy yoga classes can teach you a lot about how your body is changing, and you can learn breathing, relaxation, and movement techniques that are useful in labor.

✳ Aching sides

If your sides are aching, it might not just be down to overdoing it. Extra estrogen softens the connective tissues around your body, while progesterone relaxes your muscles and loosens ligaments and tendons.

BABIES MOVE more when you are sitting quietly, lying down, or in the bath, so if you want to feel your baby these are perfect opportunities.

GOOD TO EAT
Milk offers a bone-friendly combination of calcium and vitamins D and K.

A stretching pain in your lower belly, on one or both sides, is probably a result of the ligaments around your uterus stretching. You might also notice a jabbing or dull ache if you stand suddenly, twist, or cough. To alleviate any pain, inhale slowly, imagine oxygen nourishing those stretched ligaments, and then consciously relax the area as you exhale. Resting forward onto a cushion offers relief, too.

✳ Changing posture

Now that your belly is really growing, your center of gravity moves forward to accommodate the extra weight up front, and from your breasts, too. This exaggerates the curve in your lower back, which is further exacerbated by stretched core muscles that no longer offer support. Being aware of how you sit and stand can prevent back and neck ache later (see page 214). When sitting, whether at home or at work, place both feet flat on the floor with your thighs resting on the seat and your lower back supported to get your spine in a good alignment (an extra cushion may help). Rest your shoulder blades against the chair if you can, to open your chest and relieve shoulder tension.

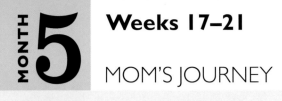

MONTH 5

Weeks 17–21

MOM'S JOURNEY

Make a dental appointment. Your risk of gum disease has increased slightly now.

Making plans

This is usually the calmest time of pregnancy, which makes it a perfect time for planning. Why not arrange a relaxing vacation as a couple, think about where to give birth, and consider your maternity leave options?

✳ Take a trip

Vacations with a baby aren't exactly relaxing—in fact, by this time next year, your notion of a vacation will feel completely warped. So make the most of this window of opportunity to enjoy one last vacation with your partner (see pages 106–107) or a group of girlfriends. Flying is easiest before 28 weeks, after which you may need a doctor's note to fly and long trips will be less comfortable. Relaxing by the coast might be more enjoyable than a hectic city break or action-packed adventure treks. Use the time to read, daydream, and talk about the future. Being away from the hassle of regular life often puts things into perspective and makes decision-making less daunting.

✳ Visit maternity units

Every mom-to-be should be informed about her options, so now is a good time to research the places you might

DID YOU KNOW?

YOUR UTERUS has now grown so high in your abdomen that it is level with your belly button!

50%

BY WEEK 20 your cardiac output (amount of blood) increases by 30–50%.

choose to give birth. Consider all the options, even if you already have a preference for a high-tech hospital or homey birthing center. You can do a huge amount of research online, and personal recommendations are also useful, but nothing beats visiting a place in person. Be ready to ask lots of questions to the staff. When visiting a hospital, take your partner with you, or a friend— preferably one who has already given birth and who will know exactly the questions to ask. Join an organized tour, or you may prefer an informal visit that might reveal a less glossy picture. While you're there, look for details of possible prenatal groups, pregnancy yoga, or relaxation classes offered on-site.

✳ Work matters

Now that everyone can see your burgeoning belly, it's time to make serious plans about when to stop work and, if you're self-employed, how to hold things together while you take time off. It's advisable to keep all your options open for the moment. You might feel sure now that you'll return to work full-time or take all your allotted leave, but you may change your mind for various reasons once the baby arrives. Some parents use this opportunity to change their working arrangements, so investigate options for part-time, job-share, and freelance work. You might even contemplate ditching your current job to set up your own business or go back to school. If you're not sure about your entitlements and options, the human resources (HR) department or union office in your workplace should be able to point you to good sources of information.

Splashing around

At this month's ultrasound, enjoy the magical sight of your baby moving around. Her muscles and joints are developing so she can stretch, turn, and kick.

✳ Growing strong muscles

While your baby was still an embryo she developed a small number of primary muscle fibers. These set the template for the secondary fibers that formed in the fetal stage. Now, these secondary fibers are increasing in mass, making the movements of the skeletal muscles— the ones she will eventually be able to control—more powerful. The movements are not yet purposeful, since the parts of the brain that control movement don't develop until early in the third trimester.

✳ Bending the knees

Developing babies don't initially have joints. The skeleton forms first as cartilage tissue, which eventually hardens into bones, but there is a space where two bones meet. In a developing baby, the points that eventually become moveable joints—the elbows, knees, neck, shoulders, hips, knuckles, thumbs, and wrists—fill with a higher density of cells, and are known as interzones. The cells at these

Baby's progress bar: you are now 50% complete

LOADING ...

10%	20%	30%	40%	50%

DID YOU KNOW?

BY 20 WEEKS your baby weighs about 8 oz (225 g). She will grow 1¼–2 in (3–5 cm) this month.

HOW BIG? Your baby is about the length of a banana.

junctions then have to "commit" to becoming part of the joint and not the surrounding cartilage. The first joint to establish itself is the knee.

✳ Working together

The muscles become increasingly active as more neural impulses are delivered to them by motor neurons in the central nervous system. This causes the muscle fibers to contract, applying force to the bones and making them move. This has a critical influence on the developing joints; the mechanical stimulation prompts the cells in the interzones to segment, with some turning into a joint rather than following the regular pathway that turns them into cartilage. The more your baby moves, the more successfully the joints will form.

✳ Varying movements

The different types of joint developing will allow your baby a full range of movement, from hinging elbows and knees forward and back to rotating sockets in the hips and shoulders.

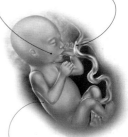

Tooth buds for milk and adult teeth are in place.

Thumb-sucking may be seen on the 20-week scan.

Spine is quite straight, with visible vertebrae.

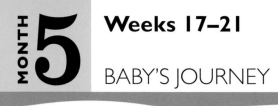

MONTH 5

Weeks 17–21

BABY'S JOURNEY

This month, your baby doubles in weight, which is mostly due to fat.

Snug as a bug

Your baby's skin is translucent at the moment, but as he starts to develop layers of fat, the skin gradually becomes more opaque. This fat will protect and keep him warm after he is born.

✳ Staying warm

While your baby is in his bath of amniotic fluid, his temperature is regulated for him, but in the outside world he'll need a good layer of fat to help him stay warm. Deposits of fatty tissue, or "brown fat," start to develop now, especially around his torso, to act as insulation. Brown fat is also an essential source of energy if your baby needs resuscitation at birth or is sick in the first days.

✳ A protective varnish

During this month a white, waxy coating develops over your baby's skin, known as vernix caseosa, a Latin term that translates literally as "cheesy varnish." That gives you a clue to its texture! This greasy covering emerges from your baby's sebaceous glands and mixes with dead skins cells, shed by your baby in the same way that our own skin constantly renews itself. Vernix protects the baby's skin from the effects of spending nine months in a bath of amniotic fluid, which contains quite concentrated fetal urine by the end of a pregnancy. Vernix also acts as a lubricant during the birth.

DID YOU KNOW?

HUMAN BABIES are the only primates to develop sweat glands over the entire body during their development.

THE SHAPE of a baby's hair follicles determines whether he has straight, wavy, or curly hair.

✳ Keeping cool

Two types of sweat gland develop this month. Eccrine sweat glands, which emit an odorless sweat, now develop on the palms of his hands and soles of his feet—by month seven, more of these glands will emerge all over your baby's body to help him cool himself. Apocrine sweat glands (responsible for smelly sweat) also start to form all over the body this month, but most of these will disappear by month seven, leaving only those under the arms, pubic area, lips, and nipples. These glands then lie in wait until puberty kicks off.

✳ Hairy baby

As early as week 12 your baby had eyebrows and lashes, then around week 16, hair follicles erupted on his scalp in a characteristic pattern, determining his future parting and the height of his hairline. By 20 weeks, a layer of fine fluffy hair—lanugo—has developed over your baby's body. No one really knows what purpose it serves: one opinion is that it helps maintain warmth; another is that it protects the layer of vernix. Hair growth begins on the upper body and moves downward, so by the time it sprouts on his legs, the hair on your baby's arms can be quite long. Don't worry—it falls off by week 36. And from week 24 "real" hair starts covering your baby's scalp.

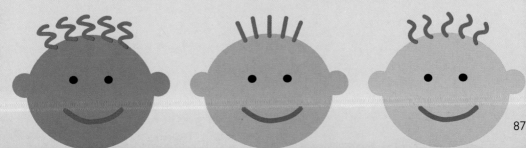

You may see your baby sucking her thumb, yawning, and stretching. She may even look a little like you!

The position of the placenta is checked.

The 20-week ultrasound

Your baby will have grown a lot since the last scan. The sonographer has several checks to make, and you might be able to find out if it's a boy or a girl.

❋ What's it for?

This detailed scan, sometimes called the anatomy scan, is usually offered between 18–22 weeks. It is primarily to see if your baby is developing and growing properly and to detect as soon as possible any physical abnormalities, such as spina bifida or heart defects. Checking two babies will take extra time! The location of the placenta is also checked; a low-lying placenta could affect your chances of a natural delivery. If this is the case you may be given another scan at 36 weeks to see if the placenta has moved up and out of the way.

If you didn't yet have an ultrasound (see page 58), this scan could give an estimated date of delivery, though it is less accurate at this gestation.

74% OF PREGNANT MOTHERS opt to find out their baby's gender from their scan, according to a 2009 UK study published in the journal *Ultrasound*.

❋ What happens?

Just like at the first ultrasound, a sonographer will put gel over your abdomen and use a handheld device linked to a computer screen to get an image of your baby.

❋ When is the due date?

A length measurement can no longer give baby's age accurately. Instead, your baby's age is estimated by taking measurements of her "bi-parietal" or head diameter, and/or the head circumference, and the length of her femur or thigh bone.

✳ Pink or blue?

At this ultrasound, the sonographer should be able to tell the baby's gender, if there is time during the scan, though whether you are told depends on whether you want to find out. Keep in mind they can occasionally get it wrong! If the baby is lying in an awkward position where it is difficult to see clearly, the sonographer will only be able to give you a best guess.

✳ What if the screen picks up something?

If your ultrasound detects a problem, the sonographer will refer you to a maternal fetal medicine specialist and also ask you to discuss the screening test with your doctor. Together, they can help parents understand risks and make decisions. In most cases, everything is just fine.

A clear picture

In the 20 week scan your baby will look even more human. She has well developed limbs, fingers, and toes, and you may even be able to make out her facial features. Her head will look disproportionately large compared with the rest of her body, just as most babies do when born. Now that your baby is bigger, she may appear to be a snugger fit in your uterus, with less room to move around in there. This can lead to her stretching her limbs while you watch.

Facial features can be seen clearly now; does she look like you?

Space is limited so baby needs to fold her limbs. This is a leg, folding at the knee.

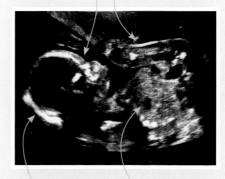

The hard bones covering the skull appear white.

The heart is checked to see if it is working well and has four chambers.

After the exhaustion and possibly the nausea of the first three months, this trimester is all about looking and feeling fantastic. Time to buy a few new clothes!

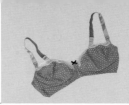

Fashion and photos—work it baby!

As your pregnancy progresses, you will find you need a few new clothes. And why not celebrate your new curves by having photos taken?

tight jeans?

You can buy maternity skinny jeans, which fit under a growing belly. Later on you might also want pants with a stretchy waistband to go over your belly so you feel warm and secure. For work, invest in well-cut pants that you can sell later.

Three tips for perfect pictures

Photos of your pregnant figure make a fantastic record of this time in your life, and will be fascinating to your child later on. You are blooming this month, so go for it!

1

Location, location, location Choose a garden, beach, professional studio, your home... anything goes. If you feel relaxed, you will probably look your best.

2

Looking good Plan the photo shoot for after you've had a haircut. Put on a little makeup and wear simple, elegant clothing, which ensures you are looking your best!

3

Lighting Flattering lighting can make a huge difference to your appearance. Choose soft, natural light if possible. The sun setting behind you can create a lovely silhouette.

YOUR BREASTS will change shape and size during pregnancy and when breast-feeding, so you will need to get fitted for new bras. Put underwire bras away for now since they can cause milk ducts to block. For now, comfort and support are the most important considerations.

Your feet and back are carrying more weight now, plus your feet may get wider for a while. If your shoes feel tight, you need to go shopping!

Your center of gravity changes when your belly is larger, making walking in high heels difficult. Make sure you can walk easily in your shoes so you won't trip.

new shoes?

Flats and low wedge heels are practical options. Shock-absorbing sneakers are great for later in your pregnancy.

It's exciting buying maternity clothes; it feels like a rite of passage to motherhood. These days you don't have to sacrifice style for comfort.

No one needs pregnancy clothes for long, so they rarely wear out. Borrow or buy secondhand, particularly for special parties or weddings.

fashion trends!

Cotton undies are the most comfortable,

Essential lists

BABY BASICS

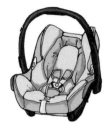

STROLLER

Can lie flat, suitable for
a sleeping newborn.

CAR SEAT

Rear-facing; removable
so you can carry baby.

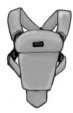

BABY CARRIER

To take baby anywhere,
and leave you hands free.

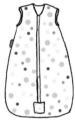

SLEEPING BAG

Keeps baby warm
without blankets.

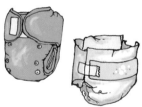

DIAPERS

Either cloth diapers (including
liners) or disposables.

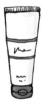

EMOLLIENT CREAM

To protect baby from
diaper rash.

BLACK-OUT BLIND

To help with restful
sleep in your room.

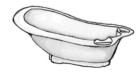

BABY BATH

Put in kitchen sink or tub;
saves water and is baby's size.

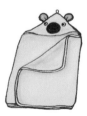

HOODED TOWEL

Soft and new, with a
hood for after bathtime.

STORES ARE FULL OF EQUIPMENT to buy, but you definitely don't need everything available: somewhere for your baby to sleep, some way of carrying him easily, and ways to keep him clean are the basics. Borrow as much as you can!

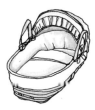

MOSES BASKET

Needs new mattress; ideal for the early weeks.

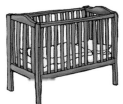

CRIB

Can be used from birth up to two years.

COTTON SHEETS

To cover the mattress of a Moses basket or crib.

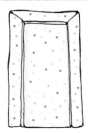

CHANGING MAT

Choose something soft and easy to clean.

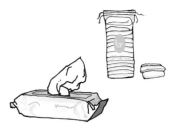

BABY WIPES

Wipes, or cotton pads, for cleaning diaper area.

BABY MONITOR

So you can hear when baby wakes up.

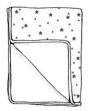

SWADDLE BLANKET

Made of cotton, for swaddling baby or to lie on.

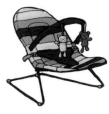

BOUNCY CHAIR

A secure place for baby to watch you.

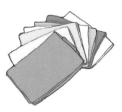

BURP CLOTHS

To protect you from drool, milk, and vomit.

The halfway mark

Your partner now looks pregnant, and it all seems very real. This month is the 20-week ultrasound where mom's and baby's progress will be checked. Your baby actually looks like a baby, and it can hit home that it's not long now.

✳ Blooming beautiful

You might think it's amazing and fascinating to see the changes to your partner's body, but some women can feel less than enthusiastic. She's probably worked hard to stay in shape over the years and now her waistline is expanding every day. If your partner is feeling dispirited, be supportive; it's a great sign that the baby is growing well.

✳ Hey girl, hey boy

Depending the baby's position, this ultrasound may bring the moment you find out whether you are having a son or a daughter. If you have decided to find out, it's best not to have any expectations. All the old wives' tales about belly size or position meaning boy or girl have no scientific basis. If you have a strong preference, you have a 50 percent chance of feeling extremely disappointed; if you stay

Do

Offer to smooth on some stretch mark cream or oil onto her growing belly every day.

Make healthy smoothies for you and your partner to boost nutrient and vitamin intake.

Continue talking to her belly so your newborn baby recognizes your familiar voice.

YOUR BABY will start to look like a miniature newborn and can hear!

YOUR PARTNER'S CENTER OF GRAVITY IS SHIFTING, SO SHE MIGHT FEEL A BIT OFF-BALANCE. A GREAT EXCUSE FOR HOLDING HANDS.

Whether you have a boy or girl will be determined by which of your sperm meets the egg.

WHY NOT START considering names? How will your ideas sound with your last name? Will the baby even have your last name? Can the name be shortened or turned into a nickname?

Don't

Make jokes about her changing shape—she is unlikely to enjoy being compared to Humpty Dumpty or Homer Simpson.

Forget to keep an open mind about your baby's gender—girls can be good at baseball, too. Chances are you won't care one way or the other when your baby arrives.

open-minded, you have a 100 percent chance of happiness. Most parents-to-be don't care whether they get a boy or a girl as long as their baby is healthy, and that is a good place to be.

✱ Checking that everything is just right

The purpose of the 20-week ultrasound is to check the development of the baby, rather than find out the sex. The sonographer will check the position of the placenta to make sure it isn't blocking the cervix, which is the baby's exit (placenta previa, see page 232). The baby's head, limbs, and abdominal circumference will be measured to find out if she is growing as expected for her age, and her spine will be checked to make sure it is aligned. The sonographer will also check how your baby's major organs, such as the lungs, heart, brain, stomach, and bowel, are growing. A repeat ultrasound may be necessary if your baby is in the wrong position to do all the checks. If there is any problem, you will be told right away and given support by professionals. Be reassured that most babies are born healthy so it is unlikely that the news will be anything other than positive.

MOM'S JOURNEY

The glowing time

Minor pregnancy complaints are usually outweighed by positives now—in addition to that beautiful belly, your hair may be thicker and glossier, and you might be developing a fabulous pregnancy "glow."

❋ Glossy hair

Estrogen encourages hair to linger in its growth phase, which makes it appear longer and in better condition. Since the strands aren't shed as fast as normal, it looks thicker, too. Make the most of this by getting a really good hair cut. You might want to make another appointment just before the birth to take you through the early days of babyhood when there's little enough time to wash hair, let alone style it!

❋ Healthy nails

Like hair, nails get stuck in a growth phase during pregnancy and can lengthen remarkably. If you're trying to avoid the toxic ingredients often used in nail polishes, opt for an old-fashioned manicure and buff your nails to boost circulation. As your belly swells and your feet get further away, consider a pedicure. Get the luxury option and treat yourself to a foot massage, which is wonderful for your circulation.

✳ Beautiful skin

Skin tends to plump up and glow in pregnancy because of all the extra circulating blood. The increased hormones encourage your skin to retain moisture, filling out fine lines, too. You are also much less likely to get pimples at this stage of your pregnancy. You might get a few tiny spider, or thread, veins on your cheeks, caused by the rapid dilation and constriction of blood vessels, but these tend to fade a few months after birth. As your belly continues to swell, your skin may begin to feel tight and stretched, so rub moisturizer or olive oil all over while your skin is damp after a bath or shower.

✳ Relaxing is essential

Retained moisture might be great for plumping cheeks, but you might find it affects your ankles and feet. You may also experience edema, also known as dropsy, when your growing belly exerts pressure on blood vessels in your pelvis, especially on the right side, causing blood to pool in the lower body. This congestion forces the extra water downward where it tries to escape through your feet. Gravity adds to this, making the effects most noticeable in the evening. Rest with your feet higher than your heart to help the blood circulate back to your heart. Lying on your left side, and doing ankle rotations, will help to boost circulation.

Naming and paying

Your baby is making herself obvious now as your belly gets bigger and her kicks get stronger. This prompts parents to think about baby names and also about who is going to take care of the baby after the birth.

✳ The name game

You might find yourselves imagining a whole little personality for your baby now, based on when and where she kicks, and how your belly is sitting. That often leads to a pet name that might be a stepping stone to a real name. If you haven't before, you might find yourself looking through baby naming sites, leaving sticky notes in books, and contemplating the expectations and associations that accompany names you are drawn to.

✳ Return to your roots

Thinking about names encourages many parents to reconnect with their own families and heritage. Names are an opportunity to make connections between families, and to celebrate the past. You may also have to confront family expectations—are you encouraged to use a first, middle, or family name that's been passed down through generations? What if you don't want to use your partner's last name? Having a baby brings together two distinct families—if you are married, you may find that naming conversations stir up as much debate as the wedding-invitation list.

DID YOU KNOW?

DADS NOW spend far more time taking care of their children. Since 1965, the average amount of time dads spend in child care has tripled in the US.

PARENTS in the US spend on average one sixth of their income on child care.

✳ Who takes care of the baby?

This is perhaps the most searching question parents have to ask as a child grows and circumstances change. After the initial newborn weeks, who will do the day-to-day child care? Will one of you take most responsibility, or will you try to share tasks? Will you call in family for help, or use a babysitter? It might be a scary option, but now is a perfect time to visit day-care centers or talk to nannies, even though you probably feel completely unprepared. The best way to find out about realistic options is to talk with parents of babies and toddlers in your area. Figure out the costs, and talk to your boss at work about flexible spending accounts, which can offer a tax break.

WHAT'S IN A NAME?

In Bali, every person has one of just four available names. A baby is named according to birth order and the names are the same for boys and girls. That certainly resolves a lot of discussion!

✳ Planning for the future

If you get maternity pay, your household salary will go down once you stop working. It's easy to push this thought away, but now is a good time to plan. Figure out how you might cut back, or accrue savings, to pay for baby items, and also about how you'll survive month-to-month. If you want to prioritize your thinking, plan for the living expenses— add up the cost of essential bills and food—and budget what's left over for vacations, clothes, and going out. On a positive note, despite what leafing through a pregnancy magazine might suggest, a newborn actually needs few essentials (see pages 92–93), and there's a huge amount of immaculate secondhand baby equipment for sale.

MONTH 6

Weeks 22–26

BABY'S JOURNEY

Your baby's brainwave patterns now start to resemble that of a newborn baby.

Starting to remember

Your baby's brain goes through a period of rapid growth at the start of this month. The cells that control conscious thought are developing, and with them, the early stages of memory.

✳ Growth spurt

Neurons proliferate while the upper part of the brain, called the cortex, grows rapidly. This growth peaks by month six or seven. As the neurons sprout transmitters and receptors to connect with other cells and send and receive signals around the body, your baby becomes more able to move with purpose and coordination.

✳ Pruning out

Brain development is not just about cell growth—any cells that are not useful now start to self-destruct. Around 90 percent of the cells in the cortex are discarded because they haven't formed the right connections, while those that have made the grade thrive and develop a protective coating of fatty material, called myelin, which speeds up the electrical impulses that pass through them. Your baby's motor reactions and senses now become more acute and efficient.

Baby's progress bar: you are now 65% complete

LOADING ...

| 10% | 20% | 30% | 40% | 50% |

BY 26 WEEKS your baby weighs about 2 lb 3 oz (1 kg) and is 11 in (29 cm) long. Your baby will grow 6 in (15 cm) this month.

HOW BIG? She is about the size of a cabbage.

✳ Startling stuff

Babies develop a startle, or Moro, reflex between weeks 24 and 28. This primitive reflex is an involuntary response to a sudden change in stimuli, such as a loud noise. You might notice your baby jump in reaction to a slammed door or car alarm. It is a fight-or-flight reaction, vital for your baby to deal with stress. Newborns are tested after birth, and show a response to noise by flinging their arms out to the sides and arching their backs. The reflex goes after about six months, replaced by a calmer reaction as your baby's nervous system matures and she learns to filter out unwanted stimuli.

Lanugo hairs keep a layer of greasy vernix on the skin, which, in turn, is starting to develop a protective outer layer of keratinized cells.

✳ New responses

Now that your baby's senses are more acute, it's no longer just your and your partner's voices she recognizes from inside the uterus. Studies suggest newborn babies recognize music they have heard in the uterus.

Daytime and nightlife

Your baby has developed a cycle of sleeping and waking, and you should be able to predict when she'll be more active—although unfortunately it might not always fit in with your own sleep schedule!

✳ Rhythm of life

Baby now starts to establish a circadian rhythm. This is the internal biological clock that governs vital body functions, such as breathing, temperature regulation, and hormonal control, over 24 hours. A master "clock" in the hypothalamus area of the brain controls other clocks in almost every body tissue to make sure that everything is working in an appropriate way for the time of day or night, and season of the year. While your baby is in the uterus, your hormones help to coordinate her own developing circadian system.

✳ What's on when?

Generally, babies seem to be most active for about five hours in the morning and again in the evening. So it is likely that you'll notice your baby moving

FROM WEEK 24 onward, your baby might survive outside the uterus if given specialized neonatal care.

32°F

Your baby's temperature is about 32°F (0.3°C) higher than your body temperature.

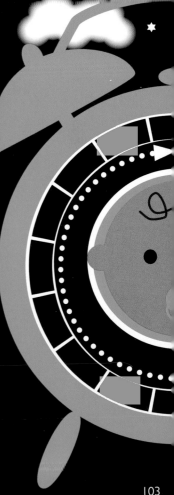

more in the evening and when you are in bed, making it seem as if she becomes more active when you are relaxing or trying to sleep.

✳ Wide awake

When your baby is in an active phase, the movements of her arms, legs, and eyes become more synchronized. Her eyes have been moving behind her sealed eyelids since about week 20, but at the end of this month, they finally open and she is able to blink.

✳ Sleeping time

Baby sleep is divided into three states: quiet, active, and indeterminate—this indicates that her brain has become more mature. Quiet sleep is similar to our Non-REM (Rapid Eye Movement) sleep, when breathing and heart rates slow. Active sleep seems to be a precursor of REM sleep, characterized by rapid eye movements, a very active brain, dreaming, and memories. Your baby spends most of her days in indeterminate sleep, which indicates that her brain is not yet able to organize activity. During the third trimester your baby will start to spend more of her sleeping time in quiet and active sleep, getting ready for her life on the outside.

6

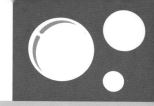

SPA IDEAS AND BEAUTY TREATMENTS

Being pregnant, you may have grooming concerns— can I still use my favorite hair dye? What products should I avoid? What are the best spa treatments for pregnant women?

Floatation tank

Unwind physically and mentally in a floatation session—you will float effortlessly in the quiet and dark, in body-temperature water. Very relaxing!

Indian head massage

If it's more comfortable to sit upright rather than lie down, try an Indian head massage, which covers your head, scalp, face, neck, upper arms, upper back, and shoulders. Research by the Institute of Indian Head Massage says it can relieve headaches, congestion, and insomnia.

Acupuncture

This can re-energize you if you are feeling tired. It can also alleviate lower back pain, and even turn a breech baby.

Facial

Pregnancy hormones can cause acne—a gentle facial may help. Facial oils can also rehydrate your skin.

Beauty treatments

Waxing, facials, pedicures, and manicures are all safe during pregnancy, though your skin might feel more sensitive than usual.

Moisturize

Use a natural, rich cream all over your body, especially on dry areas of skin, such as elbows and heels.

Haircare

In the second trimester, people might start remarking on the thick, glossy appearance of your hair (see page 96). If you usually color your hair, fear not, your routine doesn't need to change much. The chemicals in permanent and semi-permanent hair dyes are not highly toxic. But research is limited, so avoid color in the first trimester, and after that get your doctor's go-ahead. Henna dyes are safe—do a patch test first since your hair may be more absorbent.

Things to avoid

- Deep tissue and sports massages are too powerful while pregnant, even on your legs.

- Steam rooms, saunas, and jacuzzis can lower blood pressure, making you feel dizzy. Raised body temperature is dangerous for the fetus.

- Body wraps can raise your temperature, and contain chemicals that may cross the placenta.

- Tanning beds expose your skin to ultraviolet rays, which may be linked to a breakdown of folic acid. Your skin is also more likely to burn.

- Reflexology is best avoided in the first trimester, but is okay later in pregnancy.

Alternative hair dyes

If you are concerned about using permanent hair dyes, perhaps try foil-painted highlights, or switch to wash-out colorants that contain fewer active ingredients.

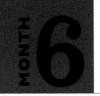

MONTH 6

Take an expensive vacation while you can before you need to pay for extra seats! Babies can travel on a parent's lap for up to two years. After that, airlines charge a full fare for children of any age.

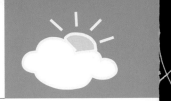

Happy babymoon

Many parents-to-be are opting to take time out to bond and relax ahead of the birth—it may be your last chance to take a trip alone for quite some time.

❋ When to go

The best time to travel is during the second trimester of pregnancy (14–27 weeks), when the waves of nausea have subsided and your belly is not yet too big. Airlines don't impose restrictions for pregnant travelers until into the third trimester, although some may request a letter from your doctor after 28 weeks.

❋ Where to go

Everyone's idea of a romantic, restful destination is different. For some, sunny beach resorts provide the perfect backdrop; for others, city breaks are preferred. Opt for somewhere with decent medical care should the need arise. Long-haul flights add unnecessary stress, as well as increasing the risk of DVT (deep vein thrombosis). Drives shouldn't be too long either and it's a good idea to take regular breaks.

❋ What to do

Nap in a hammock, lose yourself in a good book, soothe away muscle stress in the pool, or spoil yourself with a massage. Savor long, leisurely dinners together or spend the evening stargazing; take the time to bond and enjoy this special period of transition.

DID YOU KNOW?

MOVING AROUND on a long car, train, or plane trip will reduce your risk of deep vein thrombosis.

34

AFTER 34 WEEKS MOST AIRLINES WILL NOT PERMIT YOU TO TRAVEL.

A BEAUTIFUL VIEW

Traditional Chinese medicine advises looking at beautiful things during pregnancy. A text from around 290CE suggests you should "look at fine pictures, and be attended by handsome servants."

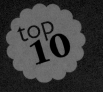

How do you do that?
GETTING A GOOD NIGHT'S SLEEP

1 ### Comfort is key
Lying on your left side can be more comfortable and aids blood flow to the placenta (so good for baby, too). Place a pillow under your belly and between your legs for added comfort.

 ### Eating habits
Try not to eat less than two hours before you go to bed, and avoid spicy and fried food. Ask your doctor if you can regularly take antacids at night.

 ### Drink in the day
Don't drink too much, or get thirsty! The recommended amount of liquid per day is eight 8 fl oz (227 ml) glasses, plus one extra glass for each hour of light activity. That includes all your intake of water, herbal tea, and soft drinks.

4 ### Enjoy some gentle exercise
If you have done some exercise, your body will be more tired and you'll feel more relaxed. Avoid exercising in the evening, though, because it can increase adrenaline, which prevents sleep.

5 ### Alarm trick
If you can't sleep, it can make you clock-watch. Try resetting your alarm for an hour later than usual since this can make you feel more relaxed if getting back to sleep takes a while. It's better to be a bit late for work than half asleep all day.

IS YOUR BELLY KEEPING YOU AWAKE, making sleep a luxury you can only dream about? Then follow these handy tips and you will soon be sleeping like a baby.

6 Dealing with worries

Having a baby gives you plenty to think about, and in the middle of the night your thoughts can spiral unchecked. If that happens and you find yourself panicking, write down what you are worrying about, then put it out of your head until morning.

7 Banish bad dreams

Pregnant women, especially with their first baby, may suffer from strange dreams and even nightmares. This is a natural result of a fear of the unknown and is normal. Relieving anxiety will help, so plan a relaxing spa treatment.

8 A soothing bedtime routine

You can practice on yourself for when the baby appears! Try hot milk, music, reading, and avoiding all screens (TV and computer) for an hour—whatever helps you wind down.

9 Nighttime baby gym

As soon as you lie down to rest it may feel like the baby inside you wakes up and starts exercising! Some people say turning on the radio can help soothe the baby to sleep again; it may also distract you from the little gymnast inside.

10 Visit your doctor

Your lack of sleep won't directly affect your baby—so don't worry. However, if it is affecting your ability to function, make an appointment to speak to your doctor for advice.

Top 10

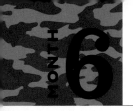

MONTH **6**

Weeks 22–26
DAD'S SURVIVAL
GUIDE

DID YOU
KNOW?

Money on your mind

It's getting very real now and it's time to start thinking about practicalities, equipment, and finances. On the plus side, you can feel baby move, too!

✳ Money, money, money

Now that you are starting to shop for your new addition, you might realize how much he is going to cost you. If you haven't already, you and your partner should figure out a budget. With one or both of you taking leave from work, you will have less money, and you will also be spending more on diapers, clothes, etc. Make time to go through your income and outflow to help avoid stress. Borrow as much baby equipment as you can, and welcome offers of gifts for big-ticket items, such as a car seat or stroller. You will probably make short-term savings by having fewer expensive nights out in the months to come.

✳ Work it baby

In the UK men are entitled to up to two weeks paternity leave, plus additional time off if your partner returns to work before the end of her

In the US there is no legal right to paid paternity or maternity leave.

ALL OF HIS SENSES are developing rapidly—he can hear low-frequency sounds, responds to light, and even has taste buds!

THE AVERAGE COST OF RAISING YOUR BABY TO 21 YEARS IS $226,920. OUCH.

maternity leave. Scandinavian countries also have good paternity benefits, but perhaps surprisingly, the US is very behind in offering any paternity leave, unpaid or not. Ask your boss or human resources manager if you can use sick time or vacation time to stay home when your baby is born. If you can take extended leave to be primary caregiver it can be a wonderful experience. It will also give you some insight into the tough job your partner does when you are at work.

✳ Move it

Your baby's movements will start to be noticeable and the nerve pathways in his ears have formed, meaning he can hear. To get a wiggle from your baby, try talking and singing to him, and you could try shining a flashlight on your partner's belly, or rest a cold drink against her if she'll let you. In the next few weeks you may be able to see baby moving as he changes position, which is really exciting and nothing for you to be fearful about.

Do

Think about taking paternity leave or time off from work.

Write down all the things you will need to track down in preparation for the baby.

Figure out a budget based on your reduced income and decide together if you will need to make any changes to your outflow.

Don't

Prod or poke the belly trying to get a reaction from your baby—you're likely to stress him out!

Put off thinking about a will or life insurance—get it done and put your mind at ease.

Whine or go out for coffee when shopping for baby items. Your input is important.

MOM'S JOURNEY

On the move

As you now enter into the final stage of your pregnancy journey, you might wonder how your body is able to accommodate your expanding baby, and where all your organs have ended up as a result.

✳ Growing belly

By week 28, the top of your uterus will be about 2½–3 in (6–8 cm) above your belly button, and from now on your belly will get noticeably higher and wider. As the baby puts on weight, your internal organs shift to accommodate this.

✳ Tummy troubles

Your stomach and intestines are squeezed upward as the baby grows, butting into your diaphragm, which increases the likelihood of indigestion and heartburn. Your intestines get squashed against your back which, along with the slowing effect of hormones, makes constipation increasingly likely, too. Both kidneys increase in length as the smooth muscle relaxes and dilates.

✳ Squashed bladder

In the first trimester, urinating was more frequent, partly due to your enlarging uterus. This problem returns now as your bladder gets squashed by your uterus, especially if your baby is head-down. Your bladder muscle has also relaxed now.

IS YOUR BABY feeling long as she stretches inside you? At seven months, she is almost the length she'll be at birth.

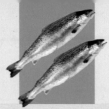

GOOD TO EAT

Oily fish with omega-3 fatty acids for development of your baby's brain, eyes, and nervous system.

✳ Opening ribs

Your ribs react to a widening uterus and higher digestive organs by expanding sideways. This can feel uncomfortably stretchy, which is exacerbated if your baby is lying head-up in the breech position.

WEIGHT GAIN slows down slightly in month seven. As your uterus presses on your belly, you feel full more quickly after meals.

✳ Breathing in

A widening rib cage affects your diaphragm. This dome-shaped muscle at the base of the lungs contracts when you inhale, moving downward to create space in the chest cavity for the lungs to expand, drawing in air. The movement is hampered by a higher uterus and stomach, so your in-breaths will feel more restricted now that the diaphragm can't move to make space.

✳ Adapting spine

The column of vertebrae in your spine adapts to accommodate the increasing weight and bulk of your uterus by exaggerating its natural curves. This can cause back pain. Postural exercises can be helpful.

✳ Cramping legs

Cramps in the legs are common from week 29, especially at night; some doctors chalk this up to increasing pressure from the extra weight straining your leg muscles, or the effect of your growing uterus on nerves in the pelvis. Shooting pains, or tingling down the backs of your legs, can be a sign that your baby's head is pressing into the sciatic nerve in the lower part of your spine.

113

MONTH **7** **Weeks 27–30**

MOM'S JOURNEY

By the end of month seven you have gained around 15 lb (7 kg).

Showers and sunshine

It's the start of a new trimester and your fast-approaching due date can feel daunting, so this is a good time to reconnect with supportive friends and family—and is an ideal time for a "baby shower."

✳ Dealing with fatigue

The energy of the second trimester starts to run out now, and it's normal to feel a little disconsolate, as if pregnancy will last forever. When your increased metabolism and squeezed organs make breathing, moving, and sleeping less easy, it's no surprise that life seems more of a chore. If you haven't done this already, figure out what tasks you can jettison or delegate at work and at home. Then try to enjoy the latter stages of being pregnant.

✳ Stress and hormones

The third trimester brings an increase in a stress hormone called corticotropin-releasing hormone (CRH), which is released from the placenta. Although CRH brings benefits to your developing baby, as a stress hormone it can have a negative impact on you. Studies show that strong family support at this time—both material and emotional —correlates to lower levels of this hormone, and fewer symptoms of depression later. This is a good time to test some of the support systems that you hope to rely on after the birth—there's still time to change plans if need be.

DID YOU KNOW?

BABY SHOWER CELEBRATIONS are traditionally intended to soothe, nurture, and shower the mother-to-be with good things.

RISING LEVELS of the stress hormone CRH (see below) help your baby's brain to develop and his lungs to mature.

✳ Pack a birth bag

Getting together everything you need for the birth can also lift a weight from your shoulders, and bring a welcome feeling of control. You might want to show your shopping list to friends planning your baby shower, and make sure you go shopping yourself before walking becomes a little difficult. In particular, consider what you might want to wear during labor, and choose some nursing tops if you plan on breast-feeding.

✳ Choice friends

You might find that some single friends aren't into the baby scene, or notice that child-free colleagues are increasingly anxious in your presence in case you go into labor. This is not the time to have additional concerns playing on your mind. Try not to take their comments personally, and spend time with more nurturing people.

✳ Start classes

This is a great time to get serious about childbirth classes—knowledge of pain-relief options, relaxation techniques, and what actually happens during labor equips you to write a birth plan (see pages 138–9), and can ease common third-trimester anxieties about delivery. These classes can be bonding experiences, too—there's nothing like practicing breath-control exercises and birthing positions to break the ice in a room of strangers! You may also meet a new set of parents-to-be who you'd like to spend time with through the remainder of your pregnancy and beyond—learning to pant and moan together has sparked many special post-pregnancy friendships.

Your baby has more than tripled in length since week 12.

Are we nearly there?

Your baby is closer to her destination—at the start of the third trimester she is lengthening and putting on weight, but there's still room to do somersaults.

✳ Tight fit

By the end of this month, your baby's movements will feel significantly stronger; her activity is building toward its peak at 32 weeks, after which space for in-utero aerobics becomes more limited. You will feel these movements as sharp kicks to the bladder or headbutts into the ribs, all of which are perfectly normal. In the past, mothers were encouraged to monitor their baby's movements, counting the number of kicks in 12-hour periods, but there's no need to record anything nowadays; just be aware of patterns and contact your doctor if the movements reduce significantly.

✳ Visible limbs

You're likely to see your belly move dramatically now, which can be somewhat unnerving. This is because your baby is getting bigger and her bones are harder (they are fully developed by week 29). It is also because your production of amniotic fluid has almost ended, resulting in reduced cushioning of limb movements.

Baby's progress bar: you are now 75% complete

LOADING ...

| 10% | 20% | 30% | 40% | 50% |

✳ Where are you, baby?

The position of kicks and visible body parts gives clues as to how your baby is positioned. At the start of this month she may be lying horizontally (known as a transverse position). By 30 weeks most babies are vertical (longitudinal), often upright with a bony skull uncomfortably wedged up into your ribs. This is also known as breech position and it is quite normal this month. Between 35–40 weeks, the presentation of your baby is very important, whether she is head-down or bottom-down in preparation for birth. The ideal position she needs to get to at the end of this trimester is head-down and facing your hip. You can help gravity along from month seven by regularly getting into a hands-and-knees position, or relaxing forward onto cushions so that the heaviest parts of your baby (her head and spine) drop into a good position for birth.

Placenta passes antibodies from you to your baby.

Brain is developing to send messages to the rest of the body.

Heart and lungs are now formed.

60%   70%   80%   90%   100%

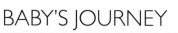

MONTH 7

Weeks 27–30

BABY'S JOURNEY

Your baby now will adopt a comfy position—arms and legs tucked up—for the duration of your pregnancy.

Getting ready to breathe

While most of your baby's body systems are relatively mature now, the lungs have some way to go before they can function after birth, so every day that goes by makes a huge difference to their development.

✳ Bigger and better

The lungs don't have to work independently until the moment your baby is born—and they spend the final trimester gearing up for this. Until last month they were completing the phase of development in which the airways branch to form bronchioles. Right now they are growing an increasing number of clusters of tiny air sacs on those bronchioles, called alveoli, which form the final subdivision of the passages inside the lungs. A network of blood vessels is forming around each of the sacs, preparing to carry oxygen from the lungs and bring back carbon dioxide to be expelled. In fact, most of a baby's alveoli form after birth, vastly increasing the surface area available for oxygen and carbon dioxide to be exchanged. This final growth phase continues up to the age of about two and a half.

✳ Super elasticity

From this month on, the smooth walls of the alveoli are receiving a very thin coating of "surfactant," an elasticating fluid that will help them to expand when they first fill with air after birth, and ensure

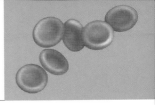

DID YOU KNOW?

THE MARROW in each of your baby's bones is producing red blood cells. In adulthood, this changes and is produced in just a few bones.

that they do not collapse when breath is exhaled. The surfactant can be detected now in your amniotic fluid. Doctors test it to find out how mature a baby's lungs are if premature birth looks likely. Rest assured, even if your baby is born prematurely, there are effective treatments that doctors can administer to help make baby's lungs more elastic.

Your baby's lungs are already praticing to inhale with amniotic fluid, rather than air.

✳ Boost that blood

Deep within your baby's bones, bone marrow is now producing most of your baby's supply of red blood cells. These cells pick up the oxygen from alveoli, via the tiny blood vessels, and carry it around the body, offloading oxygen where required and picking up carbon dioxide waste to be exhaled. The process of making red blood cells first began in the egg sac, moved to the liver, and is now in the place it will stay for life. Your baby is manufacturing fetal blood cells now, which contain the oxygen-carrying pigment hemoglobin F (HbF)— it is especially good at extracting oxygen across the placenta and combines well with oxygen from your bloodstream—it will be replaced in the last few weeks in the uterus by the adult form, called hemoglobin A (HbA). When newborn, a baby's red blood cells are up to 95 percent HbF; the remainder being HbA.

top 10

Aches, pains, and veins
COMMON COMPLAINTS IN LATE PREGNANCY

WHAT TO DO

1

Insomnia
Heartburn, needing the bathroom, your big belly… It's hard to get comfortable at night.

Be careful about what you eat and drink before you go to bed, and establish a soothing sleep routine. Sleep aids, such as pregnancy pillows, can help.

2

Numb fingers
Your fingers are numb, tingling, and you have wrist pain.

You may have carpal tunnel syndrome (see page 228). See your doctor, who may refer you to a physical therapist. Shaking your hands can help ease discomfort. Avoid activities that aggravate it.

3

Hemorrhoids
You have uncomfortable pea- or grape-sized lumps inside or sticking out of your bottom.

Hemorrhoids are often a result of constipation. Eat a high-fiber diet, drink plenty of water and fruit juice, and get regular exercise. Try not to strain when you go to the bathroom.

4

Back pain
Your lower back aches like crazy and you are starting to walk like John Wayne.

Exercise! You may not feel like it, but swimming, gentle walks, and yoga can help. Avoid standing or sitting for long periods, and if you experience severe pain or numbness contact your doctor.

5

Varicose veins
Swollen, knotty, bluish veins on your lower legs.

Avoid standing for long periods or crossing your legs. Rest with your feet and legs up, and try wearing support hose.

IT CAN FEEL like a struggle to reach the finishing line, but every day that passes brings you closer to meeting your baby.

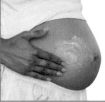

ALMOST 90% of women develop stretch marks.

WHAT TO DO

6

Stretch marks
Narrow red lines or streaks are weaving their way across your belly or breasts.

The big question is: will they go away? The answer is that they will fade to a silvery white and be far less visible. Moisturizing with oil or cream can help improve their appearance.

7

Swelling
Swollen ankles and feet, and fingers like sausages, especially at the end of the day.

Water retention in pregnancy causes this swelling. Put your feet up, wear comfortable shoes with no tight straps, and avoid standing for long periods. Remove rings if you need to.

8

Incontinence
If you laugh, sneeze, or cough you wet yourself a bit.

Increased pressure from your growing baby has an effect on your bladder control. Do Kegel exercises morning, afternoon, and night and you WILL notice results.

9

Breathlessness
You are in the middle of talking when you have to stop and pant for breath.

Sit up straight and push your shoulders back to give your lungs more room to expand. Take things easy and don't push yourself too hard when you exercise. Don't panic—it's normal.

10

Exhaustion
It's back—you feel extremely tired, all the time, again.

It's not surprising! Avoid standing for long periods or walking far (though gentle exercise can be energizing). Eat well, and rest when you need to.

Top 10

121

Essential lists

HOSPITAL BAG

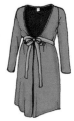

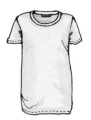

LOOSE T-SHIRT

An old, cotton T-shirt
to wear during labor.

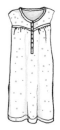

NIGHTIE

For during labor, and with
buttons for breast-feeding.

ROBE

For on the maternity unit;
don't forget a towel, too.

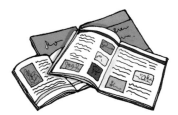

MAGAZINES

Something easy to read
during labor and after.

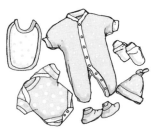

BABY CLOTHES

A few onesies, sleepsuits,
and a newborn hat.

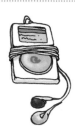

MUSIC

MP3 or CD player for
distraction during labor.

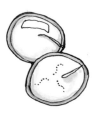

PADS

Plenty of nursing and
breast pads.

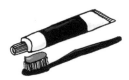

TOILETRIES

Shower gel, shampoo,
comb, and toothbrush.

YOU WILL NEED a bag for the maternity unit, including your clothes and snacks. Plan for a two day stay, though you may stay a few days longer. Your partner can pick up anything you forget, so don't worry!

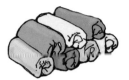

UNDERWEAR
Plenty of old, comfy or disposable underwear.

FOOD AND LIQUIDS
Tasty and easy snacks for during labor.

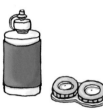

DAILY ITEMS
Any regular items you need, such as contact lens solution.

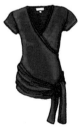

CLOTHES
For when you go home; make sure they're comfy.

EARPLUGS
For a noisy hospital; Make sure you hear your baby!

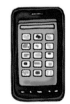

SMART PHONE
With camera and numbers you need; bring charger.

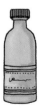

MASSAGE OIL
For your partner to give you a foot rub.

The early bird

Premature labor (before 37 weeks) can be a shock, leaving you little or no time to prepare for your baby's arrival. But although they may feel extra fragile, many early babies do not need special care.

✱ Is this it?

Your first reaction might be to panic, but try to stay calm until your doctor has assessed you—often, what are thought to be symptoms of early labor are something else. If labor is confirmed, your medical team may try to slow things down and give you steroids to mature your baby's lungs. Medical care is fantastic nowadays and babies can survive from as early as 26 weeks.

✱ Speed is of the essence

A decision may be made to induce labor or elect for a cesarean if your baby needs to come out quickly. Being induced means your labor may be faster than usual and you will be more closely monitored, so you may have to surrender some of your birth plan.

✱ A loving touch

Ideally you will enjoy a first embrace right away, but if there are immediate concerns the doctors may have to intervene, for example,

DID YOU KNOW?

FEWER THAN 20% of cases of suspected early labor result in the baby being born early. In the remainder of cases, pregnancy continues to term.

20%

if your baby needs help breathing, or if she weighs less than 4 lb 7 oz (2 kg). If she is taken to a neonatal intensive care unit (NICU), touch is especially important (see Getting involved, right). You should be able to stay with your baby day and night, but if not, ask a nurse to take a photo for your bedside.

✳ In safe hands

If your baby is born before 34 weeks, or has health concerns, she will spend time in a neonatal intensive care unit (NICU). Although it is frightening, this is the best place for her, with highly trained staff and special equipment helping her to thrive. Be patient, she will soon be coming home.

✳ Getting involved

While you can't attend to your baby's medical needs, you will play a fundamental role in taking care of her in her early days. Here are a few ways to make your time in the NICU positive for both of you.

1. Touch and stroke her—she seems so delicate, but gently stroking her can be immensely soothing and she will enjoy your familiar smell.

2. Talk to her—she already knows your voice from months inside you, so hearing you talking, singing, or just humming is reassuring.

3. Look into her eyes—holding her gaze is one of the first steps to bonding.

4. Hold her—when you are allowed to pick her up, carrying her skin-to-skin, known as kangaroo care, helps with bonding and has real benefits, actually shortening hospital stays.

5. Express your milk—this can be fed to her, providing her with immunity and super nutrition.

Entering the home stretch

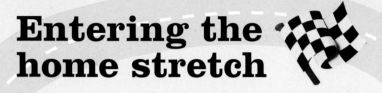

Welcome to the third trimester—the home stretch. Your partner might be getting tired of being pregnant, and there is a lot to organize.

✳ Mixed blessings

Baby will be growing rapidly, as will your partner's belly. Both of you need plenty of nutritious food, so help out by providing nourishing meals. Your partner may find it hard to sleep due to the size of her belly, and she may experience heartburn and leg cramps at night. Get used to extra pillows in the bed, and make sure she has plenty of space to move. You might need a bigger bed!

✳ Father fears

How do you feel about your partner having to go through labor? You may hate the thought of seeing her in pain, but keep in mind that labor pain is a sign that her uterine muscles are working; it doesn't mean there are problems. Maybe you're worried that something will go wrong. This is a common fear among fathers approaching the critical point, but the

YOUR PARTNER is getting achy all over. You could learn a few basic massage techniques for her head, hands, and shoulders.

MANY MEN report changes in their own sleep pattern at this point.

SOME WOMEN DEVELOP RESTLESS LEG SYNDROME NOW—REDUCING CAFFEINE CAN HELP, ALONG WITH EATING A BANANA TO AVOID CRAMPS.

IF YOUR BABY is a boy his testicles will be moving down to his groin.

chance is very low. Let's be serious for a moment: in the US these days there are only about 15 maternal deaths in every 100,000, and six infant deaths per 1,000 births. These figures are the lowest ever and continue to fall so it's good time to have a baby.

✳ Big-ticket buys

This is the time you need to bite the bullet and buy or borrow the expensive items such as a crib, stroller, and car seat. Do online research, visit stores, read product reviews, check message boards on parenting websites, and talk to parents you know. If your partner is the one who will be using the stroller most, she should be a big part of the decision-making process, even if the gadget man in you is dying to take control. It's worth buying a stroller in a store rather than online so you can see if you can both use the thing.

Do

Make sure she gets plenty of milk or another source of calcium to help your baby form his skeleton.

Feed her lots of iron-rich food to boost her production of red blood cells, and vitamin C to help iron absorption.

Take on any outstanding DIY tasks.

Don't

Panic if she experiences Braxton Hicks contractions (see page 129)—these are just practice for the real thing.

Worry about the birth. Research as much as you can so you can offer reassurance.

Forget to make your home safe, such as installing smoke alarms if you don't have them.

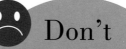

In the home stretch

Your body is the hottest it's ever been (literally), and ramping up for birth by swooshing extra blood around your system, while practicing contractions that may take your breath away.

✳ Hot stuff!

The amount of blood in your body continues to surge through your third trimester, and it hits maximum volume at 35 weeks, at around 5.25 quarts (5 liters). You have 25 percent more blood than before pregnancy and it now contains up to 50 percent more plasma (the liquid component). To deal with the extra volume, your **cardiac output**—the amount of blood your heart pumps around the body with each heartbeat—goes into overdrive. Because your blood vessels are now fully dilated, and can't relax or expand any further, they set up a resistance that causes your blood pressure to rise slightly.

✳ Can you stand the heat?

Your core body temperature has risen by almost 1.8°F (1°C) since your metabolism has speeded up, so you're more likely to sweat. Your dilated blood vessels are also working hard to cool your system and maintain a safe temperature for your baby.

NEW WORDS

- Cardiac output
- Braxton Hicks
- Oxytocin

HORMONE LEVELS are high, so you may feel elated one minute and anxious the next. Don't worry—it's your body getting ready for labor.

GOOD TO EAT
Beef for iron, B vitamins, and protein, plus chromium to support your baby's tissues.

✳ Taking the strain

All the extra fluid circulating in your body can be visible in bloated fingers and legs, as well as ankles and feet. Swollen veins may be a problem, too—blood can pool in smaller dilated veins in the lower body, such as the anus and vulva, especially as the weight of your uterus presses on the main supply veins in the pelvis. Ouch! Up to 40 percent of women notice varicose veins in pregnancy, and this tends to be hereditary. Gentle exercise and resting with your feet higher than your heart can help, as well as eating plenty of roughage, such as prunes.

✳ Let's pretend

Have you noticed your abdomen tightening and hardening from the top down? The sensation can take your breath away and tends to last about half a minute before relaxing again. This is a **Braxton Hicks** contraction, a weak, irregular version of the contractions you'll experience in labor, and a sign that your body is gearing up for the big day. The squeezing action directs blood to your placenta and starts to prepare the cervix for action. These contractions are not generally painful, but can get quite strong through the final weeks. A warm bath or back massage can help. Not all women experience Braxton Hicks contractions, however, so don't worry if you don't feel any. Your body will perform fine on the day, either way!

HOT AND GETTING HOTTER!

Building a nest

As your journey takes you closer to the main event, your body prepares you psychologically for parenthood in surprising ways. Even the least homey mothers-to-be can feel a compulsion to hang curtains.

✳ The nurturing instinct

The urge to nest reminds us of what we are in essence: mammals. Nesting is an instinct shared among mammals who give birth to offspring who can't look after themselves. For humans, it's an intuitive urge to establish a safe, sheltered place that best equips us to meet the demands of a helpless infant, and to exert a little control and calmness at a slightly uncertain time. It's best not to fight nature: give in to the urge and use it to tie up loose ends, clear the clutter, and make final decisions about how to turn your pre-baby apartment or house into a family home.

✳ Nearly time

The onset of nesting behavior seems to be triggered by **oxytocin**, the same hormone that triggers the uterus to start contracting in the first stage of labor. In fact, your doctor will be interested to hear about any extreme urge to nest in the final weeks of pregnancy, since it is often regarded as a sign that labor is imminent.

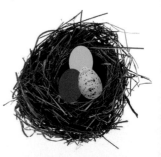

DID YOU KNOW?

MORE THAN half of dads-to-be say they experience the nesting instinct even though they don't produce the "nesting" hormone.

200

YOUR BODY will require 200 extra calories per day during the third trimester.

Although it can be tempting to balance on ladders or wield power tools as the insatiable urge to nest takes over, the more physical tasks are best left to someone else at this stage of your pregnancy. Also avoid hardcore cleaning and decorating that involves ammonia, bleach, and oil-based paints or thinners, since they give off potentially toxic fumes.

FROM THAILAND TO WEST AFRICA the birthing room is traditionally adorned with beautiful objects—beads, mirrors, painted fabric—to please the newborn baby, and deter evil spirits.

✳ Winding down

It might be sensible to figure out what aspects of your life need to start winding down. If you are working, then you will have already set your leaving date, but you may want to start delegating any new projects and handing over existing ones to colleagues. It's also a good idea to shelve any major outstanding plans, such as a moving or serious renovation work—added stress at this stage is best avoided. Instead, make time to reconnect with family and friends—they will be your primary support network in the months to come.

✳ Final plans can wait

Are you having a dilemma about whether to prepare a nursery for your baby and wondering how you'll ever have time to get it ready? Don't worry, it will be much easier to make that decision once she's here, when you'll have clearer instincts about whether she should sleep in a crib beside your bed for a while, or have her own space.

Your baby no longer needs the protection of waxy vernix or the downy lanugo hair.

Last-minute changes

At the start of this month your baby's skin still looks quite wrinkled, but by the end of the month he'll look much more like a newborn baby.

✳ Plumping up

From 30 weeks your baby will double or triple in weight, mostly due to fat. Premature babies are born wrinkled because they haven't had the benefit of these last few weeks to develop and fatten. Up to this point your baby has primarily been putting on white fat—the kind we put on as adults—which acts as a source of energy and insulator. Inside you, your baby's temperature has been perfectly regulated, kept high by your metabolism working overtime. But once outside the uterus, baby has to manage this by himself. Since newborn babies can't shiver to keep warm, they need an alternative way to generate heat. The "brown" fat laid down now helps your baby to regulate his body temperature by actively producing heat, which is carried to different parts of the body (it's the same type of fat hibernating animals use to warm themselves as they wake in spring).

BIG   *BIGGER*   *EVEN BIGGER*

Baby's progress bar: you are now 85% complete

LOADING ...

10%   20%   30%   40%   50%

DID YOU KNOW?

YOUR BABY will put on 8 oz (225 g) of weight every week throughout this month—that's more than 2 lb 4 oz (1 kg)!

HOW BIG?
He is about the size of a large butternut squash.

✳ Chubby folds

The brown fat is deposited in sheets, from the shoulder blades to the neck and down the breastbone. It continues down the arms and into the hands, creasing at the wrists and elbows to make the joints flex easily. The fat deep in the neck is particularly good at warming the blood due to its proximity to the carotid arteries.

✳ Shedding hair

The layer of fine lanugo hair covering your baby's body is now shed into the amniotic fluid. Most will disappear by birth, though you might notice traces that will fall off within a week or two after the baby is born.

✳ Soft and smooth

With this month's new layers of fat, your baby's thin skin looks less wrinkled and transparent. His true skin color will develop during the first six months after birth.

Lungs are still filled with fluid.

Pupils now dilate in response to light filtering into the uterus.

Sucking teaches baby to feed when he is born.

Weeks 31–35

BABY'S JOURNEY

A tiny teenager

The adrenal glands are getting larger and more active this month, and as a result sex hormones are triggering your baby into a phase she won't hit again until puberty.

✳ Hormone factory

The adrenal glands, positioned just above the kidneys, have almost doubled in size since month five, and are about to double again. The hormones they produce are essential for maturing the lungs, and they are working overtime right now to manufacture the hormone cortisol. Your baby needs this to trigger the production of enough surfactant to coat thousands of developing air sacs (see pages 118–119).

✳ Going into overdrive

The adrenal glands in both boys and girls also secrete huge amounts of the male sex hormone dehydroepiandrosterone. The liver processes this before it is converted into estrogen by the placenta. In addition, boy babies' testes pump out male hormones, including testosterone, which help develop the genitals. These high levels of hormones reduce after birth and are not reactivated until puberty.

✳ Birds and bees

A baby boy's testicles will probably be descending this month, dropping down from his abdomen into his scrotum. A girl's ovaries don't move into position until after birth.

YOUR BABY CAN now differentiate between sweet and sour tastes.

Women pregnant with boys eat 10% more calories than those carrying girls. Their appetite may be stimulated by hormones secreted by their babies' developing testes.

✳ Dozy baby

Also like a teenager, your baby is sleeping more this month; in fact she's out for the count for more than half the day. There's a noticeable decrease in "indeterminate" sleep and more quiet sleep now, as well as greater harmonization of her circadian rhythm (waking and sleeping times) with your own periods of rest and activity. Her sleep patterns and rhythms of day and night, activity and rest will continue to evolve during the first three to six months after birth.

✳ Beating the bugs

In preparation for life after birth, your immune system is now passing on IgG antibodies (the primary protector against invading germs and the only one of five antibodies able to cross the placenta) to your baby. You are passing on immunity against every germ you have been exposed to during your own lifetime. Sealed safely inside the uterus, your baby has been protected from germs, so her own immune system won't start making IgG antibodies until after birth; her spleen and bone marrow, however, have been producing increasing levels of IgM antibodies since the end of the first trimester.

Saving a fortune
HOW TO HAVE A BABY ON A BUDGET

Do your research

1 Find out what you really need—talk to other parents before buying tons of equipment you'll never use. Check product reviews before investing in big-ticket purchases.

Mini fashionista

2 Resist the temptation to buy designer baby clothes; babies grow out of them at an alarming rate, and often spit up on them, too! Buy a capsule wardrobe of cost-effective basics, and splurge on just one or two indulgent items. You will surely be given clothes as gifts, too.

Bargain hunter

3 Use internet auction sites to buy expensive items, such as strollers; secondhand buying can save a fortune. Save your money for things you have to buy new, such as a car seat and crib mattress.

Money wise

4 Check out any benefits or tax breaks that may be available. Look into savings accounts for your baby and put aside a little money each month, if possible.

Help from friends

5 Borrowing or inheriting from friends and family with older children can yield rich harvests of high chairs, carriers, clothes, and toys. If anyone offers to buy a gift, great—you could ask for larger-size clothes, or something specific such as a monitor.

THERE'S NO GETTING AWAY FROM IT, children are expensive. With careful budgeting and a bit of know-how you can keep the costs under control, especially in the first year.

6 Breast case scenario

Breast feeding is a great way to save money since it is free except for a few breast pads, so if you can make it work for you and your baby, that's great. When your baby moves onto solid foods you can cut costs by cooking your own baby food.

7 Diaper decisions

Diapers are a significant expenditure—to make savings consider either buying them in bulk, or using cloth diapers. The cloth route will cost you a little more in effort and laundry detergent, but your wallet and local landfill will thank you.

8 Shop smart

Buy store-brand wipes and diapers. Cotton pads are cheaper than wipes, and kinder to baby's skin, too.

9 Resale value

Unless you plan on having more children, sell anything you no longer use. Keep boxes and instructions to increase resale value and help with postage and packaging costs. Don't take labels off clothes until they get worn, so you can sell them easily.

10 Let me entertain you

Swimming and music groups are fun, but can be pricey. Check out what your local library or community center has to offer, or arrange your own informal get-togethers.

Birth plan

It's impossible, of course, to plan the exact course of your labor and delivery, but compiling a birth plan can be a helpful process as it makes you think about your options and formulate your preferences.

✳ How does a birth plan help?

This useful tool enables you to communicate with the people taking care of you throughout labor, and during possible moments when you're unable to communicate verbally. Focusing on your options and preferences for labor and birth is empowering, too, since you become informed about the process and will know what to expect. Feeling prepared makes it easier to adapt to changes on the day if events don't turn out quite as expected.

✳ What's the best approach?

You may have a vision of your perfect labor, featuring candles, a birthing pool, and some well-timed massage or, conversely, making sure that the anesthesiologist is on duty so an epidural can be administered at the earliest opportunity. The reality, though, may be quite different: events may mean a water birth proves tricky, or you may progress so fast that an epidural is not possible. Setting down your wishes is a starting point for discussion with your

DID YOU KNOW?

BIRTH PLANS were first introduced in the 1970s, and have been shown to enhance a woman's confidence during labor.

LABOR IS UNPREDICTABLE, SO A PLAN SHOULD BE FLEXIBLE.

doctor, but be aware that a birth plan is not about achieving the perfect birth or ensuring a specific outcome; it's a document stating how you intend to cope and, ideally, how you would like events to be handled.

✳ What should it include?

Think about how you want to manage the different stages of labor. Do you want to be active in the first stage, and are there positions you would like to adopt for giving birth? Would you like to labor, and maybe give birth, in water? What type of medical pain relief would you like to try, and is there anything you would like to avoid, for example, an epidural if you want to feel in control of pushing? Also, think about who you want with you during the birth. At the delivery, would your partner like to cut the cord? And do you want skin-to-skin contact with your baby right after birth, or to breast-feed immediately? You can always change your mind about any of these things on the day.

IN RURAL TANZANIA, women who are encouraged to make a birth plan are more likely to access health facilities with skilled professionals during pregnancy and in the postpartum period, giving their babies the best start in life.

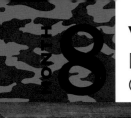
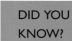
The university of life

Roll up your sleeves and put on your "bookworm" glasses; you need to do some serious preparation for the birth. Not long now, so be sure you're ready.

✳ The homework

Your partner is going to need your help in some very practical ways this month. Imagine yourself an amateur pedicurist? No? Well, you're going to need to give it your best shot just the same since she might need your help to cut her toenails. She will also be feeling tired and uncomfortable so take over her share of the household jobs.

✳ Distance learning

Practice driving the route to the hospital in bad traffic so you can time it accordingly, and know a few alternatives. If the hospital offers a guided tour, make sure you go, so you can check out what facilities are available, and so you know your way around on the big day. Find out if you are allowed to stay over night after the birth.

✳ Life lessons

It will be around now that you head to your childbirth classes, and you should go along ready to listen, make notes, ask questions, and take in as much as possible. Other dads will be there, so there is no need to

YOUR BABY gains up to half of his birth weight in the last eight weeks of pregnancy.

LOOK INTO "MEN-ONLY" CHILDBIRTH CLASSES, EXCLUSIVELY FOR DADS-TO-BE.

DRINKING MORE WATER will ease water retention, so remind your partner to drink regularly.

feel awkward. If you plan to be the birth partner (and most dads do these days) you should participate with your partner in practicing positions and breathing. It won't be embarrassing since everyone will be doing the same thing, and every piece of knowledge you gain will prepare you to be a well-informed and confident birth partner. You will be your partner's advocate on the day so you need to know what happens, what's available, and what she feels about every option, particularly pain relief.

> **MAKE SURE YOU** go to the childbirth classes whether you plan to be the birth partner or not. Be prepared for anything!

Do

Socialize with the other parents in the classes—you may make lasting friendships.

Add important numbers to your phone—doctor, hospital, and grandparents.

Drive to the hospital at different times of the day as preparation.

Don't

Make silly jokes in the classes—this won't make a good impression on anyone.

Forget everything you've learned at the classes. Practice useful positions and exercises when you get home.

Bottle up your emotions—you're not alone if you feel tense at this point.

Keep on moving

You've made it to the final month of your pregnancy journey. Hooray! Your baby can be born safely after 37 weeks, so rest easy—you're almost there.

✳ Getting comfy

Your baby is said to be "engaged" once she has dropped into a position in your pelvis where two-fifths of her head is above your pelvic bone. Once this happens you may find it easier to breathe, since your ribs and diaphragm won't feel so constricted. You'll also notice a change in the shape of your belly, which may look lower. Don't worry, however, if the head has not engaged—sometimes this doesn't happen until labor starts. You may find it less comfortable to move now; having a head wedged in your pelvis affects your posture, gait, and sleeping position. Changes also occur in your pelvis as ligaments loosen further and joints become less stable in preparation for shifting apart during birth. Many women find a pregnancy belt helpful at this stage. An all-fours position can ease lower backache: tuck your pelvis under and arch your upper back like a cat, rock backward and forward, and rotate your hips in both directions.

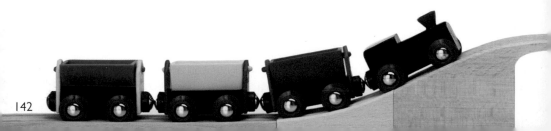

YOUR BABY DROPS deeper into your pelvic cavity this month, known as "lightening."

GOOD TO EAT
Spinach for iron and vitamin C, plus vitamin K to help blood clotting.

❋ Feeling buxom

You may notice your breasts swelling in size again as they ready themselves to produce colostrum. This thick liquid is a precursor to milk and will provide your baby with sugar, protein, and antibodies after birth, in the few days before you start making breast milk. It's normal for breasts to leak a little colostrum at this stage. Now is a good time to get fitted for a new bra to take you into the postpartum days.

❋ Practice makes perfect

In the last few weeks, Braxton Hicks contractions (see page 129) can increase in frequency, making labor seem all the more imminent. Obviously, you'll wonder if this is the beginning of labor, but if you're able to wonder about contractions they are probably not fierce enough to be the real thing! However, contact your doctor if you would like reassurance.

❋ Show time

Don't be alarmed if you notice increased vaginal discharge at this time, maybe tinted pink or brown, somewhat like the start of your period. This is a natural sign that your cervix is preparing for birth by softening and receiving an increased supply of blood. However, report any pain or bright red blood to your doctor immediately.

The final stretch

There's plenty to do during this final month, but it's important to set aside regular time each day to rest. Try to stop work with a few weeks to spare—this will help you to rest and mentally adjust.

❋ Take it easy

Last-minute shopping for baby items, cleaning the house, and planning for your new arrival are moments filled with excitement, but this natural "nesting" instinct, combined with the fact that you are at your maximum size now, can cause stress, raising your heart rate, blood pressure, blood-sugar levels, and increasing your breathing. In addition, the stress hormone cortisol will be coursing through your body at the end of the third trimester making it extra important to take it easy during this stage of your pregnancy. It's helpful to know that cortisol helps to mature your baby's brain and lungs, and can influence the time of birth; it also sharpens your senses, making you mega-attentive to your baby after birth. The downside, however, of having these stress hormones in such large volume is that you may suffer mood swings, insomnia, and reduced appetite. Progressive muscle relaxation (see Relaxation technique, right) and yoga classes can help, because they teach pregnant women how to control their breathing and how to achieve muscle relaxation (both will be useful during labor, too). Birthing hypnotherapy DVDs can also result in incredibly deep relaxation.

BE CAREFUL when going up and downstairs—
your center of gravity has now altered significantly
and you can no longer see your feet.

3–4 cm

ACTIVE LABOR is
measured from the
point when your cervix
is 3–4 cm dilated.

✳ Relaxation technique

Progressive muscle relaxation is a simple technique that teaches your
body the difference between tension and relaxation. It enables you to
tap into your body's natural responses to labor, which should help
you feel better equipped to communicate your feelings. Lie on your
left side, relaxing your top leg forward onto cushions. Inhale and
tense your right foot, lifting your leg. Hold the tension, then release
on an exhalation—let your foot flop down, and notice the relaxation.
Tense and release your calf, thighs, and buttocks. Repeat on the left
leg. Then tense and release your upper body. Finish by tensing your
face, then exhale, allowing your jaw, forehead, and tongue to
become soft and heavy. With practice you'll be able to imagine the
tension and release your whole body on an exhalation. Also try
scanning your body from the toes up. Wherever you spot
tension, picture that body part softening.

✳ Inner peace

In order for labor to start, your pituitary gland
needs to make the hormone oxytocin, which
stimulates the contractions that trigger birth.
It does this most effectively when you feel
relaxed, safe, and at ease. When tense,
you produce the stress hormone
adrenalin, which inhibits labor.
This is why many women find
contractions halt temporarily
when they reach hospital.

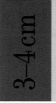

Get ready to celebrate!

By the end of your pregnancy, your large belly can be a source of sheer amazement, but you're probably ready to say goodbye to it. Buckle up, these last weeks bring you to the biggest change yet—your baby!

❋ End of an era

Labor represents an enormous emotional and physical challenge, and many women experience scary dreams and vivid nightmares during the last few weeks of their pregnancy journey. However, try not to feel too unnerved—this is a completely normal reaction to the irreversible changes your life is about to undergo—your ability to spontaneously change plans, to jump on a plane, to stay out late, or to work after hours will be curtailed when you have a baby. She will affect your relationship, too; you are a couple for a few weeks longer, then you become a family. Don't be daunted. Producing a child is the start of the best journey ever!

❋ Well-wishers

As you creep ever closer to your due date (or past it!), you are likely to be inundated with calls and texts from well-wishers. They obviously mean well, but it can be irritating to be constantly reminded that your long-awaited baby has still not arrived. If the unwanted attention is getting to you, leave a message on your cell phone explaining you'll be in touch when you have news, then switch it off.

DID YOU KNOW?

ONLY 5 PERCENT of babies arrive on their estimated date of delivery (EDD).

700

YOUR UTERUS increases 700 times in size from conception to birth.

❋ Support for the big day

You might want only your partner to be with you during the birth, but some women find that a third party, perhaps a sister or close friend, can be helpful, especially if labor is drawn out or if your partner can't get to you immediately. Discuss with your partner, and if you would like an extra birthing partner, consider who would be best suited to the task—someone you totally trust, can confide your fears in, and rely upon. Having someone who has had a good birth experience themselves is likely to increase your chances of having one, too. It's a big commitment, so show her your birth plan and perhaps take her along to a class to help her figure out her role.

❋ What did you say?

In the final weeks of pregnancy, it's common to become extremely forgetful. You'll find yourself standing in front of the fridge wondering why you're there, missing appointments, and zoning out mid-conversation. Some studies point at a reduction in brain-cell volume that affects short-term memory—it's not permanent, thank goodness. Your memory should return to normal once you're over the sleepless nights, but if the fogginess makes you feel scared or sad, tell your partner and talk to your doctor.

IN BENGAL, women in the last month of pregnancy have their every wish granted, and are given new clothes, jewelry, and fine food to prepare them for birth.

147

Ready to go

Month nine marks the beginning of the end of your pregnancy—your baby is almost ready to make her way into the world! She's putting on those final ounces and getting herself in position for her big trip.

✳ Head first

Most babies drop head-down into the pelvis after 36 weeks, tightly curled in readiness for birth. Space is limited, but you should still feel hefty kicks and jabs. If all movement stops, contact your doctor immediately. Your baby's head has been growing in circumference as the brain folds to form wrinkled troughs and peaks. The three bones of the skull are still not joined, with gaps called fontanelles in between. During labor, these spaces allow the bones to slide over each other to compress the skull and enable it to travel through the birth canal.

✳ Bring on the air

The lungs mature in the final month until your baby is finally ready to breathe air. The number of alveoli air sacs will continue to multiply and increase in diameter in the first six months after birth.

Baby's progress bar: you are now 99% complete

LOADING ...

| 10% | 20% | 30% | 40% | 50% |

DID YOU KNOW?

YOUR BABY'S head is growing ¾–1¼in (2–3 cm) per week at this stage.

HOW BIG?
She is about the size of a small watermelon.

Your baby exercises her breathing muscles by expanding and contracting the chest, and hiccupping to strengthen the diaphragm.

✳ Suck and swallow

Your baby is now equipped to process milk, and her ability to suck is well developed. Right now she's swallowing a massive 26 fl oz (750 ml) of amniotic fluid each day. As lanugo hair falls off into the amniotic fluid, she swallows that, too, along with skin cells. These lodge in the large intestine, compacting to form meconium (see page 186).

✳ Dinner on a plate

At its full size—both diameter and capacity—your placenta now weighs about one-sixth of your baby's weight, and is working hard to serve up oxygen and nutrients to the baby, and to carry waste back for you to deal with.

Skull bones are still separated for easy passage through the birth canal.

Umbilical cord is about the same length as your baby.

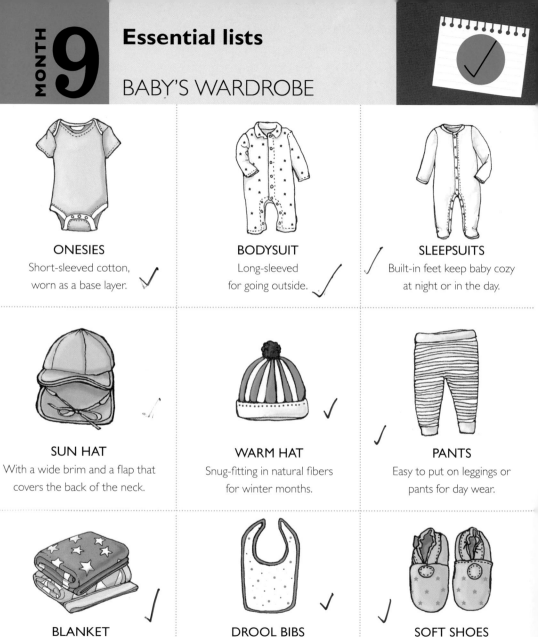

ONESIES

Short-sleeved cotton,
worn as a base layer.

BODYSUIT

Long-sleeved
for going outside.

SLEEPSUITS

Built-in feet keep baby cozy
at night or in the day.

SUN HAT

With a wide brim and a flap that
covers the back of the neck.

WARM HAT

Snug-fitting in natural fibers
for winter months.

PANTS

Easy to put on leggings or
pants for day wear.

BLANKET

For lying down on, or a
discreet feeding cover.

DROOL BIBS

To protect baby's clothes
during bottle-feeding.

SOFT SHOES

For cold weather; choose
soft leather only.

"COMFORTABLE" AND "EASY TO PUT ON" are your mantras when choosing clothes for your baby. Opt for cotton and natural fibers. Choose onesies and bodysuits with snaps, and wide, envelope necks to fit easily over the head.

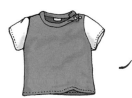

T-SHIRTS
To wear during the day over a onesie with pants.

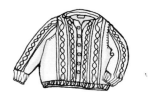

CARDIGANS
Easier than sweaters to put on and fasten.

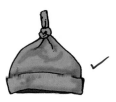

COTTON HAT
Snug-fitting for wearing outside in summer.

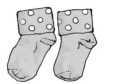

SOCKS
To keep feet warm when out and about.

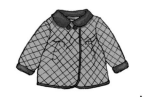

JACKET
Quilted for warmth; cotton makes it washable and practical.

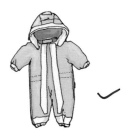

SNOWSUIT
For cold weather; always check for overheating.

SCRATCH MITTENS
To protect baby's face from sharp fingernails.

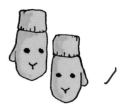

WARM MITTENS
To keep hands cosy for the winter months.

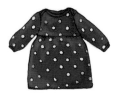

SPECIAL OUTFIT
For looking great when out and about!

Going overdue

You've reached your due date. After nine months, you're ready for labor to start, but the date comes and goes with no sign of movement. So what now?

✳ **How long can you go?**

If all is well with both you and your baby, your doctor will usually be happy to wait up to two weeks before suggesting medical intervention to kick-start labor.

✳ **What happens next?**

After 40 weeks and 10 days there's an increased risk of the placenta losing efficiency, which could affect your baby. At around 41 weeks, your doctor may offer you a membrane "sweep"—an internal examination designed to stimulate the cervix and trigger the release of hormones to kick-start labor. This increases your chance of going into natural labor in the next 48 hours by around 30 percent,

30 35 40

IN DEVELOPED COUNTRIES, as many as 25% of births are induced.

25%

Contractions brought on by the synthetic hormone syntocinon are usually stronger, longer, and more painful than natural contractions.

avoiding a medical induction. If this doesn't work, an induction will be arranged, during which drugs will trigger contractions.

The late arrival

Babies who are born late look slightly different— they tend to have long fingernails and plenty of hair, they are more alert than on-time babies, and are generally quite large.

✳ Bring it on!

If you're tired of waiting and eager to avoid an induction, you may want to try some of the following:

1. Have sex—it's thought that prostaglandins in sperm affect the cervix, encouraging it to soften and dilate. And oxytocin, the hormone that triggers labor, is released during orgasm and may stimulate contractions. It's unproven, but worth a try…

2. Nipple tweaking—if the thought of sex wears you out, stimulating your nipples is a more straightforward way to release oxytocin to trigger contractions.

3. Stay active—movement works with gravity to encourage your baby down the pelvis and put pressure on the cervix.

4. Eat spicy food—the idea is that the spices stimulate bowel muscles, in turn stimulating uterine muscles.

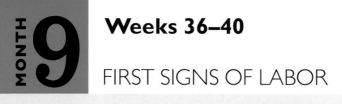

Any time now!

It's time for your baby to make an appearance, but how will you know when he's on his way? As your body gets ready to give birth, several changes happen.

✳ It's all good

Gradually, over many hours, pressure will build in your pelvis and rectum as the baby drops farther down in the pelvis, and you may develop a dull, minor backache. Although uncomfortable, these are encouraging signs that your baby is on the move.

✳ A positive sign

A bloody mucus discharge, or "bloody show," means the mucus plug that protected the uterus from infection in pregnancy has dislodged from the cervix. This can mean labor is fairly imminent, although it may be days, or more, before labor starts. Either way, it's a clear sign that your cervix is changing, getting ready for labor.

✳ The floodgates

The media portrayal of a pregnant woman's water breaking seconds before labor starts is very misleading—in only 15 percent of pregnancies does the water break before contractions have started. If it does happen before contractions start, labor is imminent and you should inform your doctor, who will want to assess you now that your baby has lost his protective seal.

THE START OF LABOR can be surprisingly hard to pinpoint
and is different for each woman. No single event signals its start; instead,
a build up of changes in your body work together to set it in motion.

✳ **This is it...**

The surest sign that labor has started is when you're having three to four strong contractions in 10 minute increments that steadily increase in intensity and duration, while the time between each one gets shorter. This is nature's way of gently managing your body's pain tolerance level. Changing position doesn't reduce the intensity, and it's pretty hard to hold a conversation during one. These true contractions start to shorten, soften, and dilate the cervix.

✳ **All systems are go**

Tempting though it may be, resist the desire to rush to the hospital at the first twinge. Being in a comfortable, familiar environment for as long as possible will help your labor progress naturally. Rest, move around, and eat when you feel hungry.

GO TO THE HOSPITAL...

- When your contractions are regular, strong, and about five minutes apart
- When your contractions last for about 45–60 seconds each time
- When your water has broken
- If you start bleeding
- If you are concerned about your baby's movement

Call in advance before setting off so the labor unit can prepare for your arrival. Don't forget your hospital bag as you dash out of the door.

IN INDIA doors in the home are left wide open during birth to mirror the "opening" of the uterus.

IN MEXICO doors are shut to keep out unwanted spirits.

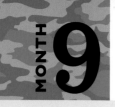

MONTH **9**

Weeks 36–40
DAD'S SURVIVAL
GUIDE

DID YOU
KNOW?

The time has come...

At last, the final month—this is the one that ends with you meeting your baby, and the start of family life. Time to brush up on your birth knowledge.

✳ On your marks...

Maybe you think pregnancy has flown by, or you may think it has taken ages. Most likely you feel both, but one thing is for sure: your baby is coming any time now whether you're ready or not! If you are the birth partner, make sure you know as much as you can about the process and the options. Does your partner want pain relief, and what does she think about, say, a water birth or vacuum delivery? Discuss the birth plan and have a copy on hand, but remember to keep an open mind and encourage her to do the same.

✳ Get set...

Earn yourself brownie points by cleaning the house and cooking a week's worth of meals to freeze. Put the car seat in now and make sure it's installed safely—you need this to bring your baby home. Your partner should have her own hospital bag prepared, but be sure you also pack key items for you: camera, sweater, snack, drink, something to read/music for waiting around, and of course your phone (fully charged) so you can give everyone the happy news. As the day approaches, check in with home on a regular basis so your partner doesn't get anxious that she can't get hold of you.

YOUR BABY will be considered full term if born any time this month.

STUDIES SHOW that women who are well supported by their birth partner have a smoother path through labor and are less likely to need intervention.

WHY NOT get a haircut now before it all gets a bit too busy.

✳ Go!

When your partner tells you she's feeling those first contractions, don't get in such a panic that you rush out of the door before you need to! For first births, it's a fairly gradual process so you probably don't need to hurry; early contractions can take days! If the contractions are spaced well apart and are infrequent, you could run a bath for your partner, or make something to eat for you both. Help your partner to stay active if she can— why not go for a short walk and make the most of the excitement of early labor. When contractions become frequent, or if you have any concerns, call your doctor's office, or the answering service if it's after hours, to report on your situation. If you are going to the hospital, wait until they give you the go-ahead, and then drive there calmly.

DISCUSS WHETHER you want to cut the umbilical cord or want a professional to do it. It's not the kind of thing you should decide on the spur of the moment.

Do

Brush up together on any positions, massage techniques, or breathing exercises you learned in childbirth classes.

Keep the car filled with enough gas to get you to the hospital, or get taxi numbers.

Load up with plenty of coins for parking or vending machines.

Don't

Spend all month waiting—make sure you both get plenty of rest, eat well, and do some enjoyable activities together.

Plan to go out drinking with friends on the eve of the due date.

Forget to buy your partner a birthing gift, and something for the baby, too.

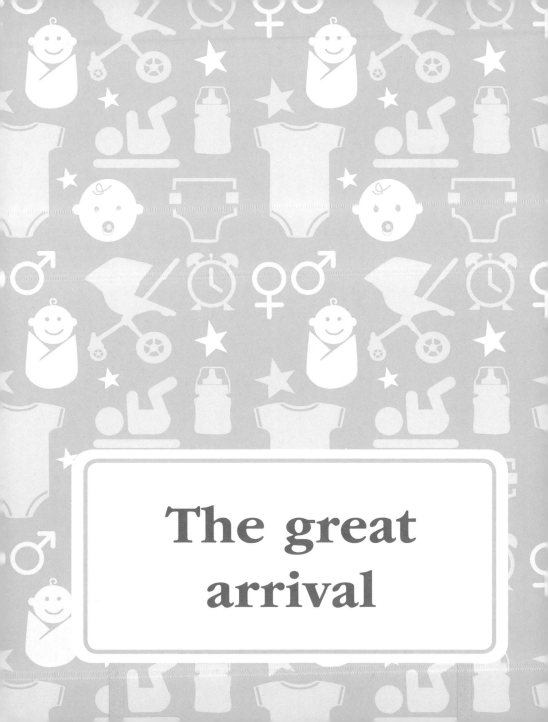

The great arrival

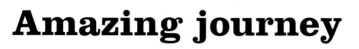

Amazing journey

Labor is one of life's greatest challenges, as well as one of its miracles. Your baby is almost with you—this is the final push!

✳ First few steps

At the beginning of labor, known as the "latent" stage, contractions are not frequent or long—maybe every 20 minutes and lasting 30–60 seconds; they are mild enough to doze or read through. As you progress into "active" labor, contractions become more frequent (every 10 minutes, then five, then two) and intense, spreading from the top of the uterus down. Each contraction lengthens to 60–90 seconds while the time between them shortens. This gets your body used to the processes of labor and increases your levels of endorphines —nature's painkiller! Leaning forward, moving around, or circling your hips can allow gravity to move the baby downward and may help. As the contractions press your baby's head into the neck of your uterus, the cervix pulls up and thins out, opening around ½ in/1 cm per hour. Finally, the cervix will draw back and your baby will pass through.

✳ On the road

The end of the first stage is called "transition"; contractions are at their most intense and frequent, with barely any time between them. This is a sign that labor is progressing well and you are about to enter the second stage—when your baby is born. The first stage transition can

REMEMBER: there is no pain between contractions, so try to focus on these breathers.

30%

DURING BIRTH you will gain 30% extra space in your pubic joint by squatting, kneeling, or being on all fours.

last for seconds or hours, as you wait for the urge to push. If you need to make noise, feel free— medical staff, and your partner, won't be fazed. If you need to have quiet around you, tell everyone to be quiet—this is your moment.

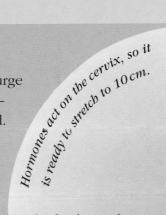

Hormones act on the cervix, so it is ready to stretch to 10 cm.

✳ The final few miles

At this stage, your baby is out of the uterus and in the birth canal. There may be a short interlude, then contractions restart, and many women have an urge to bear down, breathing deeply and working with the force of the contractions to push the baby out. For first-time moms this stage can last for up to three hours. If you don't feel the urge, your labor nurse will show you how to breathe to make the most of your contractions. Squatting during contractions aids delivery by widening the pelvis. Rest on a chair or lean forward onto the back of the bed between contractions. Finally, the head "crowns," stretching the vagina. The sensation of tingling, or burning, is intense and your doctor may encourage you to stop pushing to lessen the risk of a slight tear to the skin. First one shoulder emerges, then another, until your baby comes out and is handed to you. Well done!

✳ Almost there

The final stage is like a mini birth, only this time you deliver a soft mass of placenta, one third the size of your baby; the umbilical cord is also cut. Breast-feeding can encourage this process to happen more quickly. Your doctor may massage your belly to help your uterus contract to deliver the placenta. Delivery can take up to half an hour.

Your baby's head is said to "crown" when the widest part of his head is visible.

The final frontier

Your baby starts labor deep in the uterus with his head engaged in your pelvic brim. The minor contractions that have been gently massaging him will now push him out into the world.

✳ Ebb and flow

Each muscular squeeze of the uterine muscles contracts the uterus in size, forcing your baby down toward the neck of the uterus—the top of your baby's head has to push open the exit. This motion might break the sac of amniotic fluid, if it hasn't done before now, causing a rush of liquid—this is your water breaking. Your baby's head presses further into your cervix, which dilates until he can pass through, moving out of the uterus into the birth canal.

✳ Do the twist

As your baby descends into the pelvic cavity, he hits the pelvic floor and a slope that forces him to twist, rotating by 90 degrees. This takes advantage of the extra room between your pubic bone and the coccyx, a small triangular bone at the base of the spine, which moves out of the way. Your baby then has to rotate again to pass underneath, bending his head back so the tip of his chin leads the movement. Once this has been negotiated, the head returns to the front and his face sweeps past your pelvic floor until the crown of his head is exposed and he emerges head first followed by shoulders.

1 cm

YOUR BABY'S SKULL is, on average, ½ in (1 cm) larger in circumference than your fully open cervix. Thankfully, the bones of the skull overlap at the edges to allow the head to fit through.

CONTRACTIONS are measured from beginning to end.

✳ A safe arrival

Your baby may experience this squeezing as intensely as you—babies sometimes kick in reaction to contractions. The skull is pressured (the sliding edges of the bones protect the brain) and the placenta and umbilical cord are compressed by each contraction, reducing the amount of blood and oxygen delivered to your baby. As a result, his stress hormones are probably higher than yours. Don't worry, this serves a purpose—in a mirror image to you, your baby's stress hormones slow his heart rate and direct blood and oxygen away from his muscles toward his brain. This is a protective reaction. The hormones, called catecholamines, also trigger the lungs to step up production of surfactant, preparing the alveoli to breathe air. Your baby is monitored during birth for signs of distress, including low or high heart rates or an irregular beat. The frequency and strength of your contractions might also be recorded to see how your baby's heart responds to them.

✳ Nudging along

If your baby isn't progressing on his journey along the birth canal as expected, your doctor might break your membranes, which can speed things up, or give you a synthetic version of oxytocin by IV to make your contractions more regular. The final stage of delivery may be assisted (see pages 224–225), and your baby will be monitored continuously as he nears his destination.

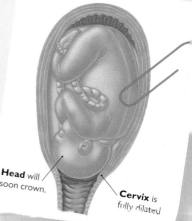

Head will soon crown.

Cervix is fully dilated

What should I expect?

LABOR IS UNPREDICTABLE

Top 10

WHAT TO EXPECT

 1 It's not time yet!

Not quite 37 weeks but contracting every 5–10 minutes for at least an hour? Had a bloody show, bleeding, or abdominal pain? Call the doctor—it's important to be assessed quickly. If your water breaks, call the hospital.

 2 Water has broken

If labor doesn't begin within 24 hours of your water breaking and you are more than 35 weeks pregnant, call your doctor to find out whether to go to the hospital. You may have to be induced because of the risk of infection.

 3 Labor just won't start

If you are very overdue, you may be offered a "sweep" (the doctor sweeps her fingers around the membranes through your cervix), amniotomy (artificial breaking of the membranes), or an induction via a stimulating suppository or induction IV.

4 Bottom or feet first

If your baby's head doesn't press into the neck of your uterus, contractions may be ineffective at stretching the cervix wide enough. For babies in breech position, your doctor may try to turn the baby, or recommend a cesarean section.

 5 Wrong way around

If your baby's back is against your spine (posterior position), contractions may be less efficient. Moving and leaning forward may help. The baby can turn once in the birth canal, or your doctor may use forceps or vacuum extraction.

ffdff

LABOR CAN START late or early, and can stop once started. It's probably best to expect the unexpected and be flexible with your birth plan at this stage...

WHAT TO EXPECT

6 **Labor is slow**

Doctors often prefer you to dilate within a set time frame and may speed things up in the first stage by breaking your membranes or giving a synthetic hormone, syntocinon. In second stage labor, you may be offered an assisted delivery.

7 **Flexible birth plan**

Planned a water birth or no medication, but it's tougher than you thought? Birth plans are great because they make you research the options and articulate what you want, but not if they make you feel stressed or guilty. Be open to all options.

8 **I need to poop!**

It's normal for you to urinate or have a bowel movement at the end of second stage—and while this may sound like the ultimate humiliation, you will neither care nor notice! Anyway, the labor nurses have seen it all before.

9 **I need to push!**

At the end of first stage, you may be ½–¾in (1–2 cm) away from full dilation but already feel the pushing urge. Pushing too early can make the cervix swell, so your labor nurse may suggest panting and getting onto your hands and knees.

10 **Checks on baby**

Some babies may need a vigorous rub to get their breathing started. Doctors will keep you informed if your baby needs any extra help in resuscitation.

A positive delivery

Think about giving birth and you're likely to imagine pushing out your baby's head: ouch! Each woman copes differently—you may find natural methods see you through, or you may need something stronger.

✳ What's a good approach?

Experiencing pain is stressful, causes tension, and impedes oxygen flow to the muscles, which then makes the pain harder to bear. It's therefore universally agreed that letting go of the fear of pain is the most positive approach to labor. The more prepared you are, knowing what to expect and how you might deal with discomfort, the more likely you are to relax and have confidence in your ability to manage.

✳ As mother nature intended

Lots of women opt for natural pain relief, either just in the early stages of labor or all the way through. There are many natural therapies (see page 226) that are effective at easing pain, have no nasty side effects, and enable you to experience every moment of your labor.

✳ Medical assistance

When natural pain relief isn't cutting it, there are various medical pain relief options that can be administered to help you deal with it. These range from drugs that help to relieve anxiety (tranquilizers), to those that block out all pain (an epidural).

IN TURKEY, from 1993–2006 the rate of women having epidurals rose from 57–96%.

In the US, epidurals are the primary form of pain relief during labor.

During the first stage of labor, contractions grow in intensity. Breathing techniques and other natural methods you've learned may carry you through most of this stage, or you may want to something like a back massage from your partner.

If you're really struggling, you can request opioid drugs or a tranquilizer, or an epidural can be put in place.

Remember to empty your bladder regularly. A full bladder can slow labor down.

Once your cervix is fully dilated and you enter the second stage of labor, it's too late for you to get an epidural. Opioids won't be given this close to the delivery since it can affect your baby's breathing. If an epidural is in place, this can be refilled.

One of the most pivotal supports during labor is that of a reliable birth partner who can help you physically and emotionally. Whether it's by your partner, a close friend, or a combination, being supported helps you deal with stress.

It is increasingly common for women to pay for a doula, a woman with training in childbirth who stays with you, supporting and guiding you throughout.

Change your position every 30 minutes, swaying in rhythm with your breathing.

Use a birthing ball, which you can lean on for support, or bounce on to encourage contractions.

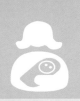

If planning a water birth at home, establish whether the floor of the room will sustain the weight of the filled pool. Make sure you have a faucet and hose nearby to fill it, and an easy way to empty it.

Water birth

Soothing, relaxing, relieving: all words we associate with warm water, so it's little surprise that many women choose to labor, and sometimes give birth, in a pool.

❋ How water helps

Immersing yourself in warm water during labor can be incredibly therapeutic. The warmth soothes muscles, releasing held-in tension, and increasing your ability to relax, which in turn helps you deal with the pain of contractions. The natural buoyancy of the water supports your weight, lifting pressure off your back and making it easier to move around and change position. It can be easier, too, to position yourself upright, such as when squatting, which enables you to work with gravity to help your baby move down the birth canal. In combination, the elements of warmth and buoyancy make for a more efficient, less tiring labor. Statistically, women who labor and give birth in water have fewer episiotomies and a shorter second stage of labor—all pretty compelling stuff!

❋ Making it happen

You can harness the soothing effects of water by simply spending part of early labor in a warm bath at home. However, if you want to use water as your main form of pain relief, and intend to give birth in a pool, check what arrangements are needed before your due date. If you're already set for a hospital birth, inquire about birthing pool

MILLIONS OF YEARS AGO the ocean's seawater shared the same salinity, 0.9%, as amniotic fluid.

5 cm

Your midwife may ask you to wait until your cervix is 5 cm dilated before getting into the pool.

facilities and whether doctors or midwives are trained in water births; if facilities are limited, see if there are birthing centers close by with pools. If you're planning a home water birth, you will need to purchase or rent a pool in advance: your midwife can give you details. You'll need a suitable space to set up the pool, where you can fill it easily, and where the midwife will have space to move around the edge. Check, too, if your midwife is experienced in water deliveries.

✳ Water slide

In a birthing center, you may not be allowed to get into the pool until you're in established labor (see pages 160–161) or until your cervix is 5 cm dilated. The water is kept at, or just below, 99.5°F (37.5°C), which ensures you don't overheat and potentially cause distress to the baby. The midwife will monitor your baby with a waterproof, handheld sonicaid, and may check how far you have dilated. If you give birth in the pool, your midwife will wait until the baby is completely delivered before lifting him to the surface for your first embrace.

THE GROWING POPULARITY of water births today has roots in 1960s France, where the obstetrician Michel Odent promoted laboring in warm water as a "gentle" birthing experience.

Your prenatal care and birth choices depend on the type of birth you are hoping for, as well as where you live and what facilities are available to you.

Home births

A home birth can offer the opportunity to give birth in familiar, comfortable surroundings and to have a greater degree of control over your birthing experience.

✳ The heart of the family

You may have known early on that you would like a home birth, or perhaps it is a decision you came to only recently. But home births are opposed by the American Medical Association and the American College of Gynecologists and Obstetricians because of the potential for complications, even in low-risk pregnancies. To be considered for one, you must have a low-risk pregnancy and no preexisting medical conditions. Being in your own home, supported by your partner and midwife, offers a familiar environment for a challenging event, and this can reduce tension, making it easier to deal with pain. You're more likely to be active, making labor more efficient: studies suggest that home births are quicker than those in the hospital. Staying in one location can also prevent a "stop-start" labor, which can happen when women move to the hospital, possibly because this interrupts the flow of hormones. Statistically you are less likely to have medical interventions or a postpartum infection.

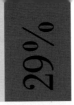

29%

✳ Getting clued in

To find a home birth provider, look for a certified nurse-midwife (CNM), a certified professional midwife (CPM), a certified midwife (CM), or an obstetrician with experience delivering babies at home. Your caregiver will have all of the essential equipment for your birth and for emergency treatment if there are complications. When you go into labor, your midwife will stay with you, monitoring your progress and your baby's heartbeat. In addition to some medical pain relief, you can use natural pain-relief methods including a water birth (see pages 168–169).

✳ Shared care

You must arrange emergency backup with a doctor or nearby hospital in case things don't go according to plan. If your baby becomes distressed or there are other complications, you'll need medical intervention.

Getting ready

Designate a "home birth" area in your home and assemble these items for the day:

- Plastic sheeting and old towels
- Bright lamp or desk light for the midwife
- Clean, warm towels and a blanket for your baby
- Any props you want, such as candles or a birthing ball

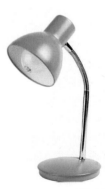

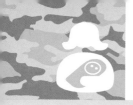

Exit via the gift shop

During your partner's labor, it may be hard to imagine that you'll look back on this as the best day of your life! But if it gets tough, remember it will all be worth it in the end.

✳ Stage One: Bring it on

As soon as your partner's contractions start, you should time both how long they last and the gaps between them. This stage can last a while so you may as well put on some music or a movie and try to relax. Make some food, even at 3 am, and stay hydrated. She may want you to run her a bath, which will help with the pain. During strong contractions, your best tactic is to stay calm and be quietly encouraging. She may want you to rub her back or try out some of the positions you learned in childbirth classes; or she may not want you to touch her at all! If seeing her in this much pain is upsetting you, just remember that every contraction brings you both closer to meeting your baby.

✳ Stage Two: Baby coming through

After some time she will feel the urge to push or be encouraged to do so by the doctor or labor nurses. Once the cervix is fully dilated it might take as long as an hour for pushing to begin. Position yourself close to your partner's head and hold her hand, telling her you know she can do it (she will be feeling pretty exhausted at this point). Remember to stay out of the way of the professionals. Don't be horrified by the sight of your squashed, slimy baby the first time you see him—this is all perfectly normal and he'll soon be looking cute. Your partner will probably want him on her chest first, but you can stay close and share his first moments.

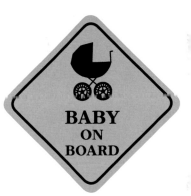

BABY ON BOARD

✳ Stage Three: You're a dad

Your partner will continue having contractions until she delivers the placenta. If she has a tear or cut, she will need stitches. Your role is no longer as simple as it was when you walked in here—you now have two people to care for. She may want you to continue holding her hand, or she may want you to follow baby's progress as he is assessed and weighed. Once everything is done, the three of you will be left alone together to recover as a family. Enjoy this precious moment before you start sharing it with the world.

Do

Take plenty of photos (nothing too graphic please).

Accept necessary changes to the birth plan—as long as the baby is safe, that is all that matters.

Cuddle your baby for the first time! Strip off and try skin-to-skin, or hold him in a towel.

Don't

Take it personally if your partner yells as you—she is in pain and doesn't mean it!

Get so distracted by keeping others up to date that you miss the birth.

Overreact if your baby is born with a birthmark. It will probably soon fade.

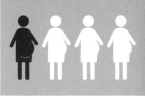

In the UK, 25 percent of women deliver by C-section, whether out of necessity or choice. The most important thing is that mom and baby arrive safely at their journey's destination.

Destination baby

The rates of cesarean (C-section) births are rising in many countries. You may want a natural or vaginal birth, but remember C-sections are usually performed when they are the safest delivery option for you and your baby.

✳ Planning ahead

A C-section is referred to as "elective" if it is planned ahead of your EDD. Usually this is because your doctor thinks it is unsafe for you or your baby to go ahead with a natural birth, for example if the baby is in a breech position, your placenta is covering the opening of your cervix, or you are expecting more than one baby. In the UK, C-sections will not be performed on maternal request in the absence of non-medical causes. If you are extremely anxious about giving birth, you may be counseled by your doctor who will highlight the risks and benefits of both modes of delivery.

✳ A change of plan

An emergency C-section is done when things do not go according to plan during a normal labor and there are risks posed to either you or your baby by continuing. This may feel like a shock, especially if you had expected to give birth naturally, but rest assured, once you have your baby safely in your arms, you will not care by what method she got there.

C-SECTIONS have been used to deliver babies for centuries, all over the world. Banana wine and botanical preparations were once considered appropriate anesthesia.

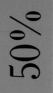

50%

IN BRAZIL half the babies are born by C-section. In Chad, this figure is just four in every 1,000 babies.

Reasons for a C-section

• Breech baby

If your baby has forgotten to turn head-down in the weeks before birth ("breech" position), your doctor may try to maneuver her by applying pressure to your abdomen. If your baby remains breech, you might be offered a C-section, although some babies turn during labor contractions.

• You have twins or more

Multiple babies can make vaginal birth more difficult if, for example, your babies share a placenta, or if one is much bigger than the other.

• Big baby, small pelvis

Very rarely, a baby's head may be too large to fit through the birth canal, so helping her out with a C-section may be the safest option.

• Placenta is playing up

A planned C-section may be safest if your placenta is lying too low, or covering your cervix ("placenta previa"), which would make birth difficult. In around one in 150 deliveries, the placenta will begin to peel away prematurely from the uterus ("placental abruption"); you may be monitored, or opt for a C-section.

• Get me out of here!

If your baby is in trouble, for example, if her heartbeat becomes irregular during labor, it may be a sign that she is not coping well with labor, and a C-section may be necessary to get her delivered as quickly as possible.

• You need to be taken care of

You may be advised to have a C-section if you have an existing medical condition, such as a heart problem or high blood pressure.

• Labor is taking forever

Despite you trying your hardest, your baby is still not coming out, and you are both really exhausted, known as "in distress." A C-section may be advised if you are not fully dilated, and have become too exhausted to continue laboring.

• Personal choice

We live in the 21st century and many women argue they should be able to choose how they give birth—be it in a birthing pool, at home, or by having a C-section. Some US doctors suggest C-sections for fear of malpractice suits with a natural birth. In the UK, most hospitals won't fund a C-section for non-medical reasons.

If you have a C-section, you may still be able to have a natural birth next time. Check with your doctor. It depends on the type of incision you had, plus personal risk factors.

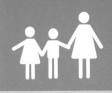

Having a C-section

Whether planned or not, going into the hospital for a cesarean section can be a little daunting—it is surgery, which carries an element of risk. Just remember that C-sections are performed every day.

✳ The nitty-gritty

A C-section is an operation where a surgeon cuts through the abdomen and uterus to deliver the baby. The cut, which falls lower than the bikini line, is made horizontally (a "transverse" incision). Vertical incisions are now rarely used since they take longer to heal.

✳ You won't feel a thing

You will be offered regional or "local" anesthesia, such as an epidural, to numb the lower half of your body. If there is time before an emergency surgery, this will also be the first option. Local anesthesia works fast, and leaves you awake to experience your baby's delivery. It also helps you recover more quickly. Occasionally, doctors may use general anesthesia, which will make you unconscious, if they think it is the quickest and safest option.

✳ Getting prepped

Surgery sounds scary, but remember your partner should be with you throughout, and at the end of it all you get to meet your baby. You will need to wear a hospital gown, and remove any jewelry or nail polish. Your pubic area will be shaved (you may be asked to do this in advance for an elective C-section), and a catheter inserted into your bladder so you don't need to worry about going to the bathroom. You will also have an IV in your hand or arm to provide medication and fluid during and after the surgery.

✳ Gently does it

You will sit on an operating table, and the table may be tilted sideways a little to take pressure off your uterus and abdomen. This is to reduce the risk of your blood pressure dropping. A screen will be placed across the lower half of your body so you can't see the surgery, but you will be able to see when your baby is lifted out. A nurse will stay near your head, and tell you what is going on, and check that you are ok. You may feel a slight tugging (like someone rummaging around in your tummy) as the surgeon lifts your baby out of the small incision, but it won't be painful.

✳ That was quick!

Your baby may be delivered as quickly as five to 10 minutes into the surgery! While you hold and get to know your baby, the surgeon will take another 30–40 minutes to remove the placenta, sew up the incision, and apply a dressing. Any scar from the surgery will eventually fade to a thin, white line that is almost invisible.

✳ Baby bonding

A nurse will make sure your baby is dried and kept warm because babies get cold quickly and operating rooms tend to be cold. Skin-to-skin contact with your baby is encouraged as soon as possible after any birth and this is possible after C-section, too. You should be able to breast-feed your baby in the recovery room soon after the surgery.

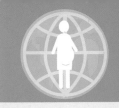

The road to recovery

You may be feeling delighted with your new baby and eager to get back to your pre-pregnancy life, but you've just had surgery, so allow yourself plenty of time to recover at your own pace.

✳ A short stay in the hospital

You will stay in the hospital for a few days to check that you have recovered fully. Your dressing will be changed after about 24 hours, and you will be given pain medication to make you comfortable as your body heals—place a pillow over your belly if you need to laugh or cough because this will ease any pain. Since you'll need to rest in bed for much of the first few days, you may need to wear support stockings (just like flight stockings) to reduce the risk of deep vein thrombosis (DVT). You are, however, encouraged to be mobile as soon as you can, and gentle activities, such as taking a shower or walking to the bathroom, will help to reduce the risk of blood clots.

✳ Gently does it!

When you get home, don't rush around trying to do everything you did before. Allow yourself time to rest, yet also try to go out and enjoy some gentle walks. Your doctor will give you advice on how to take care of your wound, to keep it clean and dry to prevent infection. You may have dissolvable stitches or you'll visit the doctor to have them removed, which takes just a few painless seconds.

YOUR PELVIC FLOOR won't have had as tough a time as during a vaginal birth. However, you still need to do your Kegel exercises!

33%

IN THE US almost one in three babies are born by C-section.

✳ Getting on with things

Your doctor and nurses will check your incision before you check out of the hospital. After that, unless you have complications, you will have a postpartum checkup with your doctor at six weeks. She will look at how your incision has healed—most women feel much better by this time. After the all-clear, many women feel well enough to get back to normal activities. Your body will get stronger month by month, but everyone is different, so take your time to recover.

🙂 Do

- Rest as much as you can, especially in the first two weeks.

- Spend time cuddling your baby. Being less mobile than usual has its advantages—you can lie on the bed or sofa with your baby and enjoy the special first days together.

- Wear large, cotton underpants and comfortable clothes to let your incision "breathe" and heal.

- Ask other people to help you with moving the carriage, making dinner, carrying laundry, or taking out the trash.

- Accept a ride, or take a taxi or public transportation, when getting out and about.

- Get gentle exercise, such as yoga or swimming, when approved by your doctor.

🙁 Don't

- Lift anything heavier than your baby for at least six weeks, since your muscles and incision are still getting back to normal.

- Forget to keep mobile—although you need to protect your incision, you also need to slowly strengthen your muscles. Keeping mobile is also important to avoid blood clots or medical complications.

- Feel guilty that you aren't able to do everything you hoped with your new baby; time spent cuddling is ideal for bonding.

- Drive in the early weeks. Your doctor may recommend that you avoid driving for two to six weeks after your C-section. Driving too soon may harm the healing process when you twist around to see behind you, or if you need to brake the car quickly.

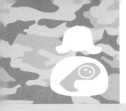

DAD'S SURVIVAL GUIDE

The road less traveled

In the US, one in three births are via cesarean section, whether planned or emergency. Obstetricians perform C-sections every day; they know what they're doing.

✳ Use an alternative route

You both may be feeling worried before the surgery, but remember you would probably be feeling pretty nervous even if your partner was having a natural birth. If your partner is having problems giving birth and the doctors have decided this is the best course of action, they will ask for her consent to proceed and she should definitely be supported in her decision. While it may not be in the birth plan for either of you, the chips are down, and the priority is getting your partner and baby safely through the day.

✳ Action stations

If possible, an epidural or local anesthesia will be used, so your partner will be awake but pain-free for the surgery. There will be a surprising number of people present, but they are all there to help the process go smoothly—this also applies to all the beeping machinery and equipment. A screen will be erected between your partner's head and abdomen, and you will stay near her head, holding her hand. A cut will be made just above her pubic bone and your baby will be handed to a nurse to dry and wrap. This will happen a few feet away and should take only a short time. Your partner will be able to hold

C-SECTION incisions heal quickly, but your partner will have stitches for at least a week.

THE BEST-LAID PLANS 40% of cesareans are planned before labor starts for medical reasons. The remaining 60% are decided during labor, for example, if the baby is getting distressed.

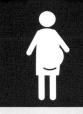

baby if she feels able, and you can help her to do this. It can take up to 40 minutes to complete the surgery now, but this is the perfect time for you both to meet your baby. Your partner can try skin-to-skin contact, which is great for encouraging breast-feeding.

✳ Recovery and moving on

After the surgery, the three of you will be moved to a recovery room. Your partner's body temperature may have dropped during the surgery, but it is nothing to worry about—the nurses will provide blankets (sometimes a hot drink) and any shivering won't last more than half an hour. Depending on the circumstances, your partner may be disappointed by the way things went—you will need to reassure her that it is not the journey but the destination that counts. Because of the incision and stitches, she may be less mobile and could find it difficult to get comfortable enough to breast-feed. Your help will be invaluable.

Do

Reassure your partner that having to depart from her birth plan doesn't matter; focus on meeting the baby.

Remember to take photos of your partner and baby. Not necessarily in the operating room, but in the recovery room and after.

Request feedback if you feel you need it.

Don't

Be afraid to ask for music in the operating room if it is calming, or have it switched off if it's not to your taste.

Watch the surgery if you know you might faint—concentrate on your partner!

Forget that your partner has had major surgery and will need time to recover.

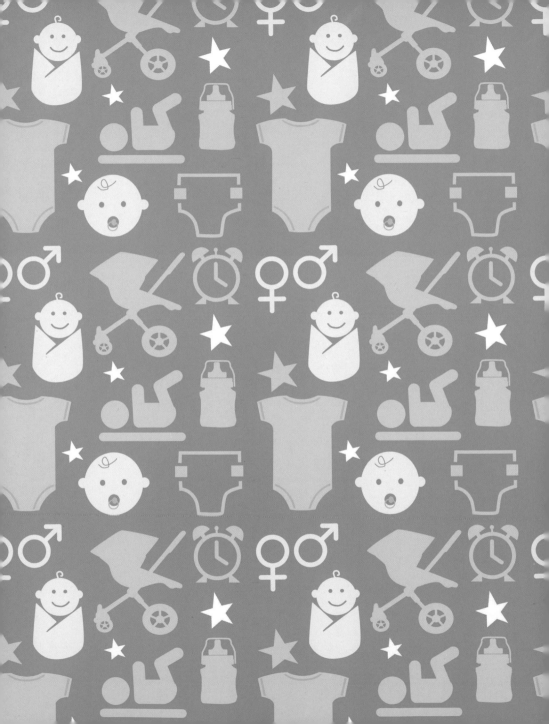

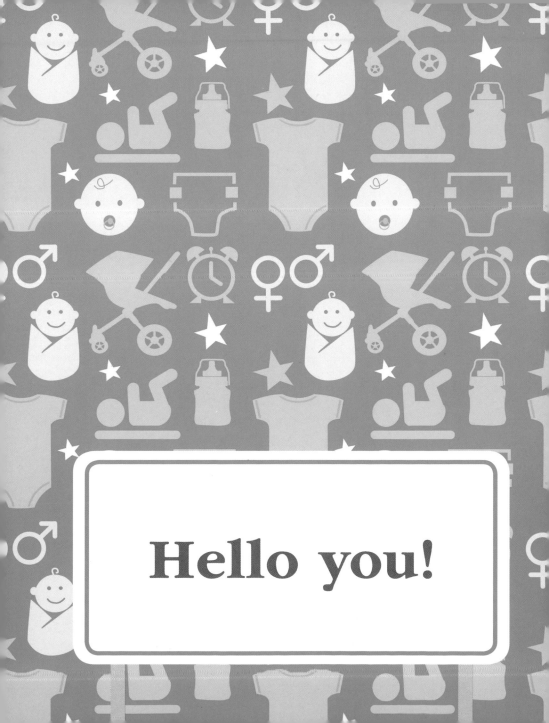

Hello you!

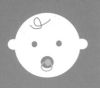

After the birth

Finally, the moment you've thought about so often has arrived—you're meeting your amazing baby! After an initial embrace, she'll need a quick medical checkup— don't worry, she'll be back before you know it.

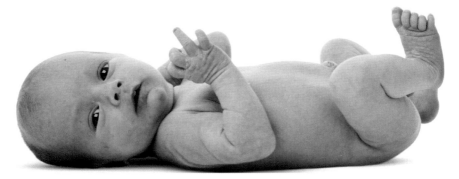

✳ Safe and sound

Within minutes of the birth, the doctor will assess your baby to make sure she doesn't need any immediate medical attention. Her pulse and breathing are checked, reflexes and skin color noted, and her movement assessed. She will also be weighed, something newborns really don't like! These tests take just a few moments and you may not even notice them happening as you recover and take everything in. You're a mom!

DID YOU KNOW?

SKIN-TO-SKIN CONTACT after birth has impressive benefits, including regulating your baby's temperature, and even reducing sensations of pain for you.

70

YOUR BABY IS BORN WITH AROUND 70 REFLEXES.

✻ Baby top-to-bottom

Within 72 hours of the birth, your baby will have a complete top-to-toe checkup (see below) to make sure all her parts are in good working order. It's most likely that she will be the picture of health, but if anything is spotted, picking it up at an early stage will ensure that help can be given quickly, and any problem rectified.

 Head The circumference will be measured and the soft spots, called fontanelles, will be checked.

 Ears It may sound odd, but the ears will be looked at to check that they're in the right position. Your baby may also be given a hearing test now, or it will be done in the first weeks.

 Eyes A light is shone in your baby's eyes to check the "red" reflex, which rules out cataracts.

 Top of the mouth The palate is checked to make sure that it is complete and the tongue moves easily.

 Heart A stethoscope is used to check the heart rate: a newborn baby's heart should beat more than 100 times per minute.

 Hands and feet Digits are counted, reflexes checked, and the position of the feet looked at to check that there's no twisting, a condition known as club foot.

 Lungs These will be listened to with a stethoscope. Breathing is checked for slow, irregular, or labored breathing, and to make sure your baby doesn't need to make an effort.

 Hips These are gently rotated (don't worry, this won't hurt) and bent to check that they aren't "clicky," a sign of dislocation or dysplasia.

 Spine Your baby will be held face-down so the doctor can have a good look at her spine to check that it is straight and there are no irregularities.

Don't panic, it's normal
THINGS NOT TO WORRY ABOUT WITH YOUR NEWBORN

1 ### Black poop
Newborn babies produce a very dark, olive-green poop called meconium. The color and texture of your baby's poop will progress to yellow and brown as he takes in more milk.

2 ### Spitting up or vomiting
Babies often throw up a small amount, or even a large amount, of their feeding. It's likely due to gas, but if it's shocking and projectile, take baby to the doctor. As long as your baby keeps down most of his feeding and is gaining weight, don't worry.

3 ### Milk spots
Around 40 percent of newborns develop tiny whitish pimples on their face, neck, and scalp. These milk spots, called milia, are caused by the sweat and oil-secreting glands springing into action. Don't be tempted to squeeze them; they will disappear.

4 ### Mysterious blotches
Raised, red blotches can appear almost anywhere on your newborn baby's body and are another harmless result of sweat and oil glands starting to work. The condition will almost always disappear within the first four or five days.

5 ### Is that dandruff?
Cradle cap looks like crusty scales on the scalp. Don't pick or poke at it since baby's skin is sensitive; it will disappear on its own. Gently rub olive oil into his scalp then shampoo it off.

SPOTS, BLOTCHES, AND BLACK POOP can all be slightly alarming if you're not forewarned. Here are ten things your newborn baby won't be worrying about, and neither should you.

Scaly skin

6 Dry, flaky skin is common, especially in overdue babies. Keep bathing to a minimum—one bath a week should be enough—and rub olive oil or baby moisturizer into his skin afterward.

Mongolian blue spot

7 Large blue marks on a baby's bottom or lower back are very common in babies of native American, African, Asian, or Hispanic descent. They are totally harmless and disappear within a year or so.

Pulsing fontanelle

8 Your baby's skull bones are not yet knitted together, allowing his head to fit down the birth canal more easily. The soft part at the front is called the fontanelle and may pulsate in time with his heartbeat—this is normal (if a little unsettling!).

Stork marks

9 Around half of all babies are born with small areas of redness on the nape of the neck, forehead, or eyelids. These are known as stork marks and will eventually fade away to nothing, though it can take up to a couple of years.

Blood in a girl's diaper

10 During pregnancy, high hormone levels can stimulate a baby girl's uterus to shed a tiny amount of blood within the first week of life. A smear of blood in her diaper is nothing to worry about.

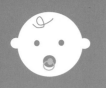

All Caucasian newborn babies have blue eyes, while newborns of African or Asian descent have dark gray to brown eyes. Their final eye color won't be set until six to nine months.

YOUR BABY MAY CRY, BUT HE WON'T SHED TEARS UNTIL HE IS ONE TO THREE MONTHS OLD.

Newborns in a nutshell

Over the following days and weeks, you and your partner can spend time getting to know your new baby—prepare for an emotional roller coaster!

✳ Love at first sight?

Bonding with your baby follows its own timetable, so enjoy the journey. You may experience an overwhelming sense of love and emotion at the birth, or you may feel exhausted. Sometimes the joy, or shock, of having a baby only hits you when you get home from the hospital. Remember, there is no "right" way to feel, because everyone responds differently.

✳ Babies can look funny

Your baby may have a cone-shaped head, be red and wrinkly, or dry and scaly—don't worry, this is all perfectly normal. It's amazing how quickly a baby's skin and head shape change after the birth. Take guidance on taking care of your newborn from nurses and doctors. Ask plenty of questions; the more you know, the more confident you will feel. Soon you will be at home without their help, getting on with being a wonderful parent!

Mama!

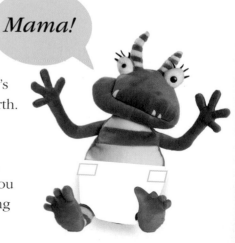

DID YOU KNOW?

NEWBORNS BREATHE around 40 times per minute. An adult breathes in and out between 12–20 times per minute.

UNDER SIX WEEKS, A BABY CAN FOCUS ONLY 8–12 IN (20–30 CM) AWAY.

✳ The first six weeks

Leaving the hospital can be nerve-wracking, so accept all offers of help. Then once at home, you can focus on your baby. For the first six to eight weeks, some newborns sleep most of the day (see pages 196–7). You may find it hard to manage if your baby is more wakeful at night than in the day, but he is born with a set of skills to help him get your attention, and to encourage you to take care of him. The easy days will become more frequent as your baby grows. And then, at about six weeks, you will be blown away when he first smiles.

IN ARMENIA,
it's customary for women to remain in the house for 40 days after the birth. Only those in the household can see the baby.

NEPALESE FAMILIES take their newborn to a priest to choose the name.

SURVIVAL **TACTICS**

1. Being born is thirsty work and your baby will want to be fed with milk soon after.

2. Within one hour of being born, your baby needs to be fed every two to three hours. Don't worry about setting your alarm for every feeding —he will let you know by crying.

3. A newborn loses five to eight percent of his birth weight within the first week, but should gain it back quickly.

4. Newborns can be noisy sleepers. Don't worry if he snuffles, snores, and hiccups.

5. If you are breast-feeding, get as much help and advice from experts as you can.

6. If bottle-feeding, have some packaged ready-made formula available as back up, but don't make up a feeding too far in advance.

7. Your baby will poop several times a day and urinate every one to three hours, though less often if breast-fed. Change his diaper to avoid a rash.

8. It's amazing how time-consuming a newborn baby can be, so any help with cooking or cleaning should be accepted gratefully.

9. Refer to pages 150–1 for your baby's wardrobe list. Having a supply of clean clothes and diapers on hand is a life saver.

189

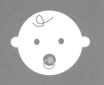

Breast milk is the right food for your baby; nothing can replicate it exactly. However, breast-feeding doesn't work for every new mom, which is when formula makes sense.

Breast-feeding or bottle-feeding?

Breast milk is the ideal first food for your little one. But why is this, and does it mean that your baby misses out if breast-feeding isn't for you?

✳ Why breast-feed?

• Your milk adapts constantly as your baby's needs change. From the nutrient-packed "pre-milk," known as colostrum, which is produced at birth, to the higher-fat, calorie-dense milk that comes through several days later, its composition evolves to ensure your baby grows and thrives.

• Breast milk boosts immunity, too, providing antibodies and white blood cells that protect your baby in the first vulnerable weeks and months. This is something that can't be replicated in formula.

• Breast-fed babies have fewer ear infections, respiratory problems, and eczema than bottle-fed babies.

• Breast-feeding is a smart system of supply-and-demand—as your baby sucks, nerve endings in your breasts are stimulated, triggering the release of the hormone prolactin, which signals your body to make more milk. You should always produce exactly the right amount of milk for your baby.

• Breast milk is thirst quenching, as well as filling. At the beginning of a feeding, your baby enjoys more watery "foremilk," and as your breasts empty, richer, fattier "hindmilk" is released.

• Moms benefit, too. Breast-feeding triggers the release of the hormone oxytocin, which causes your uterus to contract after birth. Combined with the calories used, many women report rapid weight loss. Longer term, breast-feeding may lower your risk of various cancers and osteoporosis in later life, too.

• Breast milk is easier to digest than formula, and babies are less likely to be constipated.

• It's convenient; you can feed your baby anywhere, producing milk at the right temperature.

• Breast milk can help to stimulate your baby in the daytime and relax her at nighttime.

THE FIRST FORMULA was developed in 1867 and has evolved over the years, with many companies investing in research.

1867

5 BEST BURPING TACTICS

1. Hold your baby upright, her head over your shoulder, and rub her back in a circular motion.

2. Sit her on your lap, supporting her in an upright position, and lean her forward slightly while rubbing her back.

3. Lie her face-down across your lap, supporting her securely under the arms with one hand while you rub her back.

4. Lie her down on her back and rotate her legs back and forth in a cycling motion.

5. Cradle her face-downward along your forearm, supporting her head with your hand, and rub her back while gently swinging her.

✳ Why bottle-feed?

• If you decide to bottle-feed, you can be confident that formula, derived from cow's milk, provides a high-quality alternative to breast milk. Designed to replicate breast milk as closely as possible, formula meets all your baby's nutritional needs. Choose a formula with more whey protein since it is easier for your baby to digest.

• It can be reassuring to know exactly how much milk your baby is drinking.

• Bottle-fed babies have steadier, more predictable weight gain than breast-fed babies. There is a variety of bottle sizes, so you can match the bottle to your baby's appetite, but make sure you don't overfeed her.

• You can share the experience with your partner and take turns doing night feedings to get a little more sleep.

• There are no sore nipples, embarrassing leaks, or worries about whether what you eat and drink will affect your baby.

IN 2010,
79 percent of new moms in the US breast-fed their babies after birth.

THE US, FRANCE,
Italy, and Spain have the highest rates worldwide of bottle-fed babies.

Feeding your baby
GREAT TIPS FOR BREAST-FEEDING

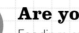

A lactation consultant can help you get started.

1 Are you sitting comfortably?
Feedings can last from ten minutes to an hour, so sit comfortably with your back well-supported. Place baby on a U-shaped feeding cushion, or pillow, so your arms don't get tired.

2 Gather everything you need
Have a glass of water (to replenish fluids), a book, your phone, or the TV control on hand since feeding may take a while. Then when your baby is latched on, sit back and try to relax.

3 Is baby ready?
Gently stroke your baby's cheek with the back of your fingers to trigger her rooting reflex, which makes her open her mouth and turn, or "root," for your nipple.

4 Latch on
Getting your baby to latch on is the key to easy feeding. Place her nose opposite your nipple; when she opens her mouth, bring her toward you. She should take the areola (dark area around your nipple) as well as the nipple into her mouth and start drinking.

5 Take your time
Leave her on your breast until she has finished, so she gets both the watery hydrating "foremilk" at the start of a feeding through to the thicker, nutrient-dense "hindmilk." Then change breasts.

BREAST-FEEDING is simple once you've mastered it, but it can be tricky when you first get started.

MOST MOMS produce more milk through their right breast, but you must use both!

Go with the flow

6 Young babies need to be fed at least every two to three hours since their tiny tummies hold only a little milk. Feeding on demand is best for your baby and your milk supply.

Wear a maternity bra

7 Your breasts will feel uncomfortably full at times, so a supportive bra is essential. A clip or zip opens the cups for quick access!

Sore nipples?

8 Air your breasts between feedings if you can, and apply lanolin-based nipple cream to soothe.

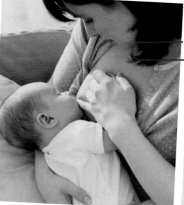

Sore breasts?

9 If your breasts become engorged, feeding can relieve fullness. It shouldn't last long.

Keep going!

10 The first few days, or weeks, can be challenging, but once you've got the hang of it breast-feeding provides instant food for your baby anywhere.

193

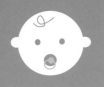

Ways to soothe baby

WHY IS HE CRYING?

CRYING IS OFTEN
MORE FREQUENT
in the late afternoon
and early evening.

Hush little baby

Hearing your newborn baby cry can be distressing, especially if you aren't sure what is wrong. As you get to know your baby you will soon find out why he is crying and learn how to soothe him.

❋ Rock-a-bye baby

Even if you're not sure what's wrong, holding him will always be welcomed. Pop him in a baby carrier and gently bounce or walk around—this usually helps. Or, try driving him around the block or taking him out for a walk in a carriage; the motion is soothing.

❋ Keep calm and carry on

Babies can pick up on stressed vibes, so keeping calm is important. If incessant crying is getting to you, take him out of the house: a change of scene will do you both good. If you are really starting to lose it, put your baby down in a safe place and let him cry for five minutes while you leave the room, take deep breaths, and remind yourself that "this will pass." Look at the checklist, right, for signs of why your baby might be crying.

The length of time a baby spends crying increases until about six weeks after birth, followed by a gradual decrease in crying until three to four months. After that, crying remains relatively stable.

VOICES
Sing or talk to your baby in a low, calm voice.

WHITE NOISE
Turn on a ceiling fan, hair dryer, or static radio.

BATHING
Some babies love baths, even in the middle of the day.

BARE UP
Snuggle your baby against your bare skin and heart beat.

Soothing solutions

SUCKING
Offer a pacifier, or a clean finger or knuckle.

PHONE A FRIEND
Go on a visit or invite a friend over.

FRESH AIR
Go outside.

CRYING CHECKLIST

Hungry? Smacking lips, rooting, eating hands—Feed

Tired? Yawning, avoids eye contact—Sleep

Dirty diaper? Check and change

Wants to be held? Calms when picked up—Pick up and hold

Tummy trouble? Crying after a meal, knees pulled up—Gas

Too cold? Cold torso—Change clothes or wrap in a blanket

Too hot? Red and sweating—Strip off a layer of clothing

Wants less stimulation? Passed around a lot, loud noise—Sleep

Wants more stimulation? Been doing the same thing for a while—Play

Teething? Red cheeks, hard nub of a tooth breaking through—Rub on teething gel

Not feeling well? Diaper rash, temperature, a cold or cough   Take temperature

RUN THROUGH this list to see if you can figure out what's upsetting your crying baby—then act accordingly.

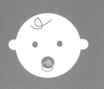

Newborns sleep for an average of 16½ hours per day, evenly divided between day and night. By three months he should sleep for about ten hours at night, breaking for feedings, and five in the day.

Blissful sleep

You may also be astonished by how much a newborn sleeps, and it can be weeks before he figures out day and night. For the first few weeks let your baby dictate proceedings, and then move toward a routine.

✳ Soothing space

A baby's brain slowly learns to distinguish day from night. Keep night feedings as restful as you can in order not to wake your baby too much. If you need a light on, make it dim and keep him wrapped up—you're both more likely to get back to sleep if warm and relaxed. Don't bother changing him, unless his diaper is dirty, and no talking.

✳ Where to sleep

For the first six months it's safest for baby to share your room in a bassinet or crib—babies learn to roll over very young, making a bed or sofa risky. Place your baby on his back to sleep, in pajamas and a baby sleeping bag. Loose blankets aren't allowed, but a thin one is okay if you: place your baby's feet at the crib's bottom; tuck the blanket securely under the mattress's bottom and sides; cover the baby only to chest height; and don't overheat the

DID YOU KNOW?

THE IDEAL POSITION to lie your baby during daytime naps is flat, rather than in a car seat or stroller, but don't worry about keeping too quiet or darkening the room.

A MOSES BASKET OR BASINET IS IDEAL FOR YOUR NEWBORN.

room—64.4°F (18°C) is ideal. Current advice is to avoid co-sleeping (sharing a bed), but if you do, you need to know that babies who live in a home with a smoker, or who share a bed with someone who drinks alcohol, takes drugs, or is on medication (these all interfere with normal sleep patterns) are at most risk. Never sleep with a baby who was born prematurely or had a low birth weight. If you choose to co-sleep, keep pillows and covers to a minimum.

✳ What to wear

Baby sleeping bags are popular across northern Europe, preventing infants from pulling covers over their heads or sliding beneath blankets. In the summer, or in hot climates, dress your baby lightly and check for overheating by feeling his tummy.

✳ Bedtime routine

Putting a baby to bed in the same place, around the same time of day, builds associations between bedtime and rest. Bedtime routines work from around three months; maybe try a bath followed by massage, then a feeding with soothing music. Place your baby in his crib while sleepy, but not exhausted, so he can drift off on his own. Try to avoid rocking your baby to sleep and then laying him down: babies who fall asleep in mom's arms can find waking alone in a different place disorienting and they may need to be settled again.

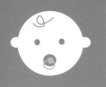

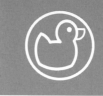

A bath cushion is a great piece of equipment to have if you are nervous about holding your baby and washing her at the same time. There are several styles and designs available on the market.

Bathtime!

Babies don't need a daily bath—a quick "sponge bath" will do. But some love bathtime so much that it turns into playtime, and on days when you both feel tired, there's nothing more soothing than a shared dip.

✳ How to bathe a new baby

You will need a baby bath or plastic bowl, a soft, clean baby washcloth, cotton pads, and a soft, hooded towel. You don't need shampoo or baby bath products for tiny babies, though you can use them if you want. Make sure the room is warm and your baby is alert and happy. Why not try quiet baby background music?

1. Half-fill the baby bath with lukewarm water (around between 95°F and 100°F). Undress your baby to her onesie and diaper. It's easiest to do this on a soft towel placed over a changing mat on the floor.

2. Moisten a cotton pad and carefully wipe one eye from the center outward (babies often have gunky eyes). Wipe the other eye using a new cotton pad. Repeat around the ears and nostrils, if necessary. Be firm but don't press too hard on your baby's delicate skin.

3. Soak a baby washcloth, squeeze out most of the excess water, and wipe her face gently, avoiding her eyes. Then wipe around her neck creases where milk and sweat can build up and cause dirt and irritation. Pat dry with a warmed towel.

4. To freshen her hair, hold your baby with her head supported by your hand or the crook of your arm, above the bathwater. Scoop water over the hair until any cradle cap is washed away. You don't need baby shampoo every time. Pat dry.

DID YOU KNOW?

IN TURKEY, MOTHER AND BABY are traditionally taken to the hammam baths on the 40th day after birth for a celebration of ritual cleansing, song, and feasting.

IT'S GOOD TO BATHE HER BEFORE HER LAST FEEDING OF THE DAY.

✳ Sharing a bath

Some babies hate being naked. If this is the case for your baby, try bathing together. Step into the bath and check the temperature is lukewarm (body temperature). Have your partner pass you the baby, cupping the back of her head and bottom. Rest her back against your chest, her bottom in your lap to support her. When ready to get out, pass the baby to your partner before getting out yourself.

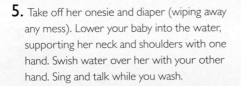

5. Take off her onesie and diaper (wiping away any mess). Lower your baby into the water, supporting her neck and shoulders with one hand. Swish water over her with your other hand. Sing and talk while you wash.

6. Uncurl her fingers to clean her hands. Wash beneath her arms and clean around her bottom. Lift her out, supporting her head and bottom, and wrap her in a warm towel. Pat dry, rub lotion into dry skin, and put on a clean diaper and clothes.

CAUTION: Never leave a baby in the bath alone, even for a few seconds.

New mom's survival guide

PLAN YOUR DAY

1 **Carrier!**

Babies love being held by both their parents, and enjoy the closeness and safety. Carrying your baby in a baby carrier when out and about can be enjoyable and avoids having to take a carriage everywhere you go.

2 **Day tripper**

When feeling cooped up at home, make plans to go out for the day, perhaps to meet up with a friend or relative who lives farther afield. If you're nervous about going on a bus or train, travel by car or take someone with you on the first trip.

3 **Cultural stimulation**

Your newborn baby may sleep for hours in the daytime, so take advantage of this down time and go out and do some of the things you never normally have time for—visiting museums, galleries, or a local attraction.

4 **Me time**

Being a new mom is wonderful, but you also need time to yourself in order to stay sane. Plan for your partner to take care of the baby one night while you spend some time with your friends. You can still enjoy a glass of wine even if you are breast-feeding.

5 **Meet and greet**

Most first-time moms will be experiencing the same emotions so it is a great time to connect with new people. Invite postpartum friends over for coffee or out to a baby event, such as daytime "baby" screenings at your local movie theater.

IT'S GREAT FUN BEING a new mom, but it can also be daunting. Here are a few hints and tips on moving on to parenthood, and enjoying life with your new baby.

6 Regain your shape

The nine-month wait is over and your baby has been born—but you still look pregnant! Now could be the time to start exercising and eating healthily in order to regain your figure. Don't diet if breast-feeding, however, since this may affect your milk production.

7 Feeling blue

Most new moms will feel very emotional during this hormonally turbulent time and for some this can turn into baby blues, or even postpartum depression. Talk to your partner about your feelings, or seek help from a professional.

8 Baby classes

Sign up for mother-and-baby classes since they are a great way to meet first-time moms like yourself. Try baby yoga or massage, fitness and swimming classes, or baby music time. Both you and your baby will love it!

9 Bonding

You may feel that you are running around all the time and need a rest. Take time out just to stay at home and hold your baby; let him touch your skin and gaze into your eyes, because this bonding has a very positive effect for both him and you.

10 Work-life balance

Although you may not be using them at the moment, don't forget that your work skills and interests are still there—you are just taking a break. Don't feel guilty about not working; being a new mom is wonderful but it is still a tough job!

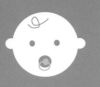

Baby blues

DOWN AT HEART

Taking care of you

Babies are wonderful, but they need a lot of care—and so do new moms. Your hormones are still all over the place, and fatigue can make you wonder where "the old you" has gone.

✻ Those pesky hormones

Remember what your body has achieved: you have successfully created a new person, and now you are trying to get back a sense of normalcy. But your hormones are running amok, so it's really common for new moms to get "baby blues" a few days after the birth. It is thought to be caused by a huge drop in estrogen and can make you feel overwhelmed with emotions. Baby blues can peak three to 10 days

Do

Read upbeat magazines and books to keep you entertained when your baby is sleeping.

Stock up on healthy snacks that are quick and easy to eat, such as fruit, muesli, and nuts.

Give yourself a mood-boost, such as visiting a beautiful place.

Don't

Feel you have to invite every member of the family over—you are still recovering.

Watch the news: take a break from depressing stories for a while.

Soldier on in silence. If you are feeling exhausted, anxious, or just not yourself, tell your doctor.

A GLASS OF BUBBLY to celebrate the arrival of your baby is just what the doctor ordered, but if you are feeling depressed, drinking more won't help.

ONE IN SIX new moms has an episode of the "baby blues."

after birth (see below if you feel down or overwhelmed longer than that). Sleep can really help so if you can, get someone to take care of your baby so you can catch up on rest—you will feel much better.

✳ Sharing the load

Perhaps more than at any other time of your life, right now you need TLC, nutritious food, and sleep—but with a newborn to take care of that is a tall order! Welcome all the help you can from your partner, friends, or family. Perhaps your partner can be in charge of putting your baby down at night or making dinner. Maybe a friend can sit with your baby while you take a bath. Get groceries delivered; hire a cleaning person; ask someone to walk the dog. If you are used to being with work colleagues, then suddenly the day can seem quiet, even with a new baby in the room. Invite people over and don't worry about suggesting a time limit if you need to rest. Even if you don't feel hugely social, at least try to get out every day and talk to people. There are plenty of parent-and-baby groups to go to; try as many as you can to find which you enjoy the most.

✳ Something more serious?

If life feels overwhelming, or if you experience any of the following symptoms, talk to your doctor for advice:

- Finding it hard to see the funny side of things
- Feeling lonely and bored
- Crying and feeling overwhelmed
- Getting scatterbrained; showing up late and forgetting things
- Finding it hard to sleep even when you are really tired

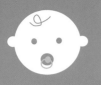

The six-week checkup

FOR YOU AND YOUR BABY

Your postpartum checkup

Your doctor will check that your body has recovered from the delivery, and that you are managing the sleep deprivation and the new-mom hormonal roller coaster. After a number of routine checks (see below), you will be completely done with your pregnancy-related office visits.

Urine test

Prepare to urinate in a cup. A urine test ensures you don't have an infection (it's okay to admit to leaks, and feeling scared to have a bowel movement). You may also be reminded to do your Kegel exercises.

Weight and blood pressure

If you are unsure about the best diet for breast-feeding or losing baby weight, ask. You might have questions about starting to exercise (if you can find time).

Abdomen and pelvis

The doctor will check that your uterus has contracted and any cesarean scar, tear, or episiotomy has healed. An internal examination

shows whether your cervix has closed. You'll be asked about your discharge (mention anything heavy, smelly, or painful), and be advised when to have a Pap smear.

Breast check

Ask the doctor to check your breasts if you are worried about anything, whether breast-feeding or not. Milk ducts can easily get blocked.

The sex question

Try not to laugh too much when asked about contraception. Lack of sleep, squirty boobs, and a baby in the room may mean sex is the last thing on your mind, but some women are pregnant at their six-week check. You can be fertile again before your periods start!

TIME TO GO OUT In many cultures women stay at home for a while after the birth, but by six weeks—if you haven't already—it's time to venture out into the world and show off your new baby.

Your mental health

How are you coping generally? It's not shameful to admit to bouts of crying or rage against your new lifestyle (see pages 202–3). Sleep deprivation makes everyone feel terrible.

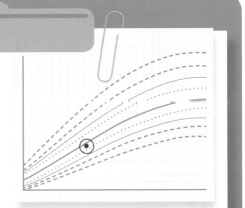

Your baby's checkup

This takes places separately, at the pediatrician's office, six to eight weeks after birth. It's a good time to ask about feeding, vaccinations, and anything that's concerning you. You'll be asked to undress your baby for weighing.

Weighing and measuring

Your baby's length, weight, and head circumference are plotted on a graph in your child's medical chart. Some pediatricians write down the numbers for you to take home. Don't worry if your baby isn't on a specific percentile (growth measurement)—not everyone is average. The key is that he's growing.

Reflexes and muscle tone

The doctor checks that your baby can hold his head in line with his body and balance his head when pulled to a sitting position. Reflexes in the eyes are also checked.

Body systems

Your baby's heart, lungs, head, spine, ears, eyes, palate, hips, legs, and genitals are all checked for development. The doctor will check for signs of inherited problems, such as congenital heart disease, hip dysplasia, glaucoma, or cataracts. Boy babies are checked to ensure that their testes have descended into the scrotum.

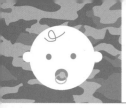

A whole new world

You've made it home with your brand-new baby. Welcome to this uncharted territory, full of unfamiliar sights, sounds, and smells. Have no fear—you will soon learn the customs and feel completely at home.

✳ Trying to sleep

As comfortable as your bed may be, you will inevitably find getting a good night's sleep a challenge at first, so grab any opportunity for 40 winks. If Grandma arrives and offers to do some housework or take your baby for a stroll, say yes, and snuggle into bed with your partner for a power nap. Don't drink endless cups of coffee to help you stay awake or it will be harder to snatch that bit of sleep when you can. Remember though, your partner is more tired than you, so fill a bottle with formula or expressed milk and give her the precious gift of a few hours of undisturbed sleep.

✳ What to do all day

Your partner will be busy taking care of the baby, as well as recovering from the delivery, so you need to take care of her. If she is breast-feeding, get her cushions, a beverage, and the remote control. Once your baby is fed she can hand him to you, the new resident burping expert. Burping is a good technique to learn and it means that your baby will get to know your sounds and smells and become bonded to you. You could also take charge of baths for the

YOUR BABY will make a swimming motion with her arms and legs if she is placed in water. This is a survival reflex and doesn't mean she's an Olympic hopeful. Don't try this without holding her firmly!

71% **OF PARENTS** and babies across the world co-sleep (see pages 196–197).

🙂 Do

Take responsibility for a couple of aspects of the baby care.

_____

Leave work on time and cut back on commitments temporarily to give you and your family time to acclimatize.

_____

Arrange for food to be delivered each week from an online supermarket.

🙁 Don't

Be too hard on yourself—it'll take time to learn the skills and demands of fatherhood.

_____

Feel down about your loss of sleep and leisure time—this doesn't last forever!

_____

Assume your partner knows all the answers; you are on this strange journey together!

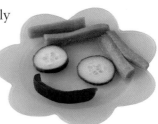

time being—having a regular routine will help your baby settle in and feel happier, and it's a good way to get quality time together. Cut back on your exercise regimen and other commitments temporarily, but take the time to relax by going out for a walk or gentle jog. If possible, rearrange your work schedule or take some leave—spending time at home now will mean you can help establish routines. Offer to take the baby out in her carrier and your partner can have a break while you're gone. It's a great opportunity to get out and show off your baby.

✱ What's on the menu?

Keeping yourself and your partner well-fed is likely to be your responsibility, so make time for nutritious meals and plenty of water. You don't need to be a five-star chef, but producing something edible will earn you major hero points. Once back at work, eat healthily at lunch to take care of yourself, too.

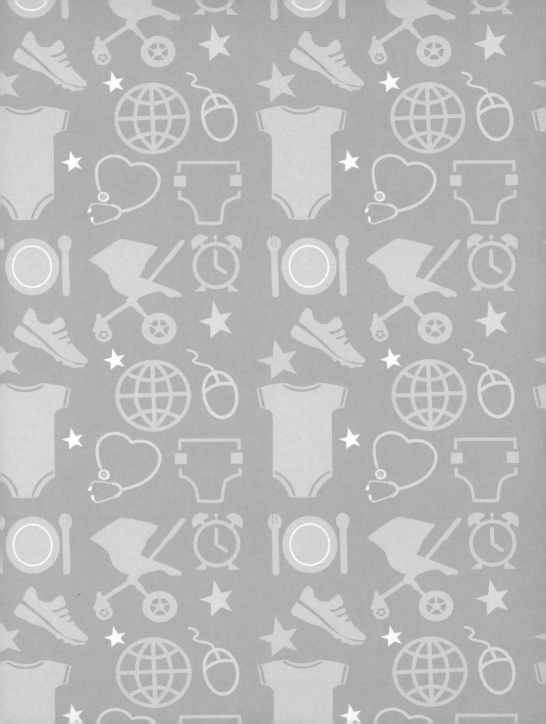

Quick reference guide

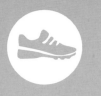

EXERCISE

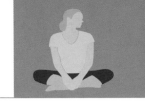

Figuring out your workout

Many people think of pregnancy as a time for taking it easy, but while rest is important, you need to make sure you are fit and well for the journey ahead.

Rest is best?

The changes in your body during pregnancy can put it under enormous strain, and giving birth is one of the most physically demanding things you will ever do. Your path through labor and delivery is likely to be smoother if you feel fit and strong. You do also need to rest, and if you take part in a lot of exercise, you might need to listen to your body and rest more.

Body benefits

Regular cardiovascular exercise will help you keep your weight gain from going too far above the average (25–35 pounds/10–12kg). It also boosts the function of body systems such as your circulation and digestion, which are under pressure at this time. Gentle exercise, such as swimming and yoga, can help prevent problems with joints and tendons. What's more, maintaining a good level of fitness during your pregnancy will make it easier to get back into shape once baby is born.

Making adaptations

It is possible to exercise throughout your pregnancy and in most cases there is no real need to change your usual regimen. You can run, dance, and cycle, though common sense and your doctor would suggest you minimize your risk of falls by switching to a stationary bike or running machine. If you feel like your body is telling you to stop or slow down, then listen to it. If you are a gym regular, get a new gym program that suits your

TOP TIP

CAN YOU STILL TALK? You should be able to hold a conversation when exercising. If you become too breathless to talk then your activity is too strenuous.

20% **INCREASE IN HEART RATE** during pregnancy equals that of low-level aerobic exercise.

body, and switch to lighter weights. Contact sports, such as basketball and karate, or any sport where you could fall (such as horse riding or skiing), should be put on hold. If you don't have a regular exercise plan, you can put one into action while pregnant, but discuss it with your doctor first.

Walk, swim, and stretch

Cardiovascular activity, such as brisk walking or swimming three or four times a week, reaps real benefits. You may find your energy levels improve and you sleep better at night. Just 30 minutes of brisk walking or swimming will be effective. Swimming is usually safe throughout pregnancy, and the sense of weightlessness can be a real tonic when gravity is no longer a friend. Yoga and Pilates are ideally suited to pregnancy as they combine relaxation and stretching with core-strengthening movements that target the muscles that are under the most strain in pregnancy. Seek classes specifically for pregnant women.

Do

- Stay active every day, even if just walking. Try for at least 30 minutes most days.

- Tell the instructors of any classes you attend that you are pregnant. There may be safe variations you can try.

- Learn exercises to strengthen your pelvic floor (see page 215).

- Find a yoga, Pilates, or pool-aerobics class for pregnant women. You'll be able to exercise safely and meet other expectant mothers.

Don't

- Stop exercising. Find exercise that feels good, safe, and keeps you active.

- Forget to listen to your body; if you start to feel nauseous or dizzy take a break.

- Exhaust yourself—you may have to tone down the intensity of your usual exercise routine; your body will give you clues!

- Do anything too strenuous in hot weather or allow yourself to become dehydrated.

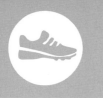

Gentle strengthening

STRONG CORE MUSCLES are vital during pregnancy since they support your spine and help you maintain the correct posture.

Exercises First trimester

These toning and stretching exercises are designed to develop the muscles you use most in everyday life and need to be strong during pregnancy: your core abdominals, thighs, and glutes (buttocks).

1

CORE STRENGTH Inhale, and as you slowly exhale push your lower back down until it is flat on the floor. Hold the position for five seconds, then repeat eight times.

2

FLEXIBILITY STRETCH Take hold of your toes. Inhale, and exhale as you lean forward for a gentle stretch down the back of your leg.

3

LUNGE Stand with your feet hip-width apart, and step one leg forward. Lower toward the floor, then return to the start. Repeat eight times, then change to the other leg.

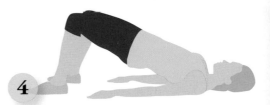

4

BRIDGE Raise your hips, bring your knees together, while tensing your buttocks. Open and close your knees 10 times before slowly lowering your hips.

Move to improve

FEELING BETTER? If initial nausea has settled down, use this time to stay active with three gentle cardiovascular activities each week, such as swimming or walking.

Exercises Second trimester

Energy levels are higher in the second trimester, so these exercises are more dynamic. You are advised not to exercise on your back after the first trimester.

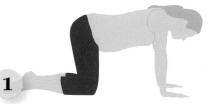

THE SLING Inhale, and as you exhale draw your muscles up and in toward your back, as if lifting your belly. Gently return to the starting position and repeat 20 times.

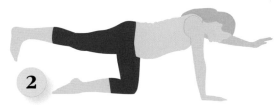

SUPERMOM Lift your left arm and right leg and hold for a count of five while still breathing. Lower slowly and repeat on the other side. Repeat on both sides eight times.

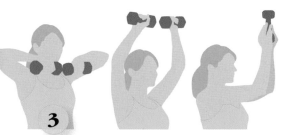

UPRIGHT ROW Inhale, and exhale as you raise your weights (4 lb [2 kg] each) slowly above your head. Bring your elbows together, then apart again. Inhale as you lower slowly. Repeat 16 times.

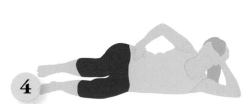

LEG IT Lift and lower your top leg slowly, without raising it above hip level. Repeat 30 times. Turn over to repeat on the other leg. Add a pillow under your belly as support if you feel like you need it.

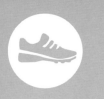
Exercises Third trimester

Your changed body shape and an increase in fatigue can affect your mobility and balance. Check your posture and keep your back strong and supple.

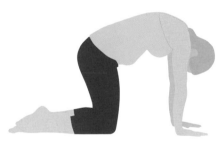

ENJOY A CAT STRETCH Your hard-working back will benefit from a gentle daily stretch. This exercise will also activate your abdominal muscles. Inhale as you pull in your abdomen and round out your back. Let your head and neck relax gently downward. Hold this position for five seconds, while breathing and without locking your elbows. Exhale as you flatten your back. Repeat eight times.

THE IMPORTANCE OF GOOD POSTURE

Good posture will help remove the stress on your back.

SHOULDERS Relax your shoulders and try not to let them hunch forward.

BACK Keep your back straight and don't be tempted to exaggerate its curve.

HIPS When standing, keep hips square and bottom tucked in.

KNEES These should be soft when standing and you should avoid crossing them when sitting.

FEET Keep your feet hip-width apart and flat on the floor when standing or sitting.

STRONG LEGS will prepare you for beneficial labor positions, such as squatting and staying mobile when you are tired.

ONE-IN-THREE WOMEN experience some pelvic floor weakness during or after pregnancy, such as stress incontinence. Simple exercises can help avoid this. You can do them any time, any place!

Don't ignore your pelvic floor

Your pelvic floor is a muscle that stretches like a sling from your pubic bone to the base of your spine, holding your bladder in place and controlling urine flow. Pregnancy can weaken your pelvic floor, leading to stress incontinence and reduced sensitivity during sex. Building pelvic floor strength with Kegel exercises in pregnancy can help prevent development of these issues.

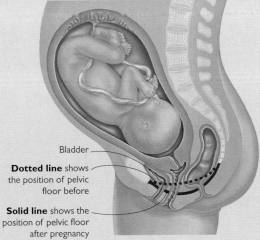

Bladder

Dotted line shows the position of pelvic floor before

Solid line shows the position of pelvic floor after pregnancy

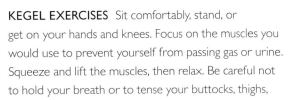

KEGEL EXERCISES Sit comfortably, stand, or get on your hands and knees. Focus on the muscles you would use to prevent yourself from passing gas or urine. Squeeze and lift the muscles, then relax. Be careful not to hold your breath or to tense your buttocks, thighs, or stomach as you lift. Once you get used to the feeling, try holding for a few seconds at a time. Repeat 15 times. Add more squeezes each week. Continue this during and after pregnancy to maintain your strength.

215

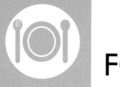

FOOD

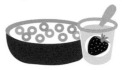

Breakfast

We all know that breakfast is "the most important meal of the day," and this really is true during pregnancy. By morning you haven't eaten for eight hours or so, and you need to break this fast.

If you are feeling sick in the mornings, or you are in the habit of skipping breakfast, then you need to find some simple, appealing ideas that you can introduce into your daily routine. Try for as much variety as possible—maybe one morning you will have time to cook a simple breakfast, such as poached eggs and bacon. Other days, a bowl of cereal or toast will be all you have time or appetite for. To make this important meal as nutritious as possible, choose whole-grain breads and cereals. Many cereals are loaded with sugar, so if you can make your own muesli or granola on the weekend to eat during the week, you can omit the unwanted sugars.

• Oatmeal can be very soothing to a turbulent tummy. Measure out the oats the night before, and pour water or your choice of milk (cow, soy, or almond are all good options) over, so the oats are well soaked by morning. Simply heat through in a pot and stir for three minutes or until the oatmeal is ready. Top with dried or fresh, chopped fruit.

FIBER AIDS NUTRIENT ABSORPTION and will help keep your blood-sugar levels steady. Roughage is easily available at breakfast time with whole-wheat toast and cereal. Try for 1–1½ oz (25–30 g) of fiber per day.

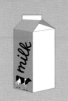

TWO SERVINGS of dairy products every day give you the calcium you need.

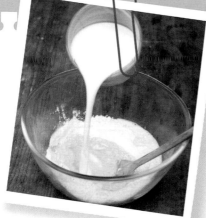

Crepes

MAKES ABOUT 6 CREPES

If you are not feeling great, crepes are easy to digest.
Mix together to form a batter:

4½ oz (125 g) all-purpose flour
pinch of salt
1 egg
1–1¼ cups of milk

Cook for 2–4 minutes, turning once.

• Bake a batch of muffins using whole-wheat flour. Add any combination of flavors, such as sunflower seeds, dried fruits, nuts, and dried or fresh berries.

• Eggs make a quick and nutritious breakfast. Buy free-range eggs that are omega-3 enriched. Serve with toasted seeded bread for extra vitamin C and fiber. Stir in frozen, chopped spinach while cooking.

• Keep a selection of rye, seeded, and whole-wheat breads and bagels in the freezer. Top with avocado, nut butter, cream cheese, or low-fat cheese instead of jam.

• Make a smoothie. Blend a handful of frozen berries, a chopped ripe banana, and 4 fl oz (100 ml) yogurt or milk.

• To make your own muesli, mix oats and wheat flakes, dried apricots, sunflower seeds, and almonds.

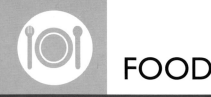
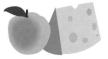

Main meals

If your appetite is affected by your pregnancy, or you prefer smaller meals at the moment, go for variety and pack in plenty of nutritious ingredients.

When planning your meals, go for a variety of ingredients so you and your baby get everything you could possibly need— carbohydrates, proteins, and fats—this is not the time to cut anything out (see pages 30–1 for more information). Think about ways you can add plenty of vegetables to every meal: frozen, canned, and fresh all count!

Try to eat at least three different types of vegetables every day, and two or more fruit. If you are feeling tired, don't think you have to cook a hot meal every day; a substantial salad or soup packed with beans and vegetables would give you everything your body needs. On days when you, or your partner, have energy, cook extra food so you have meals

in the freezer for the days when you're too tired to cook or for after your baby is born. Pasta sauce, lasagne, chicken pot pie, roasted vegetables, and stews all freeze well. Include brightly colored fruit and vegetables because they contain vitamin C and carotene, which may increase the production of infection-fighting white blood cells to prevent viruses.

YOUR BABY can taste what you eat from an early stage—strongly flavored foods can be tasted in amniotic fluid.

50% OF YOUR FOOD SHOULD COME FROM CARBOHYDRATES.

Asparagus, broccoli, and ginger stir-fry

A quick and easy meal to boost iron, and to help alleviate nausea. Add a portion of protein, such as cashews, tofu, chicken, turkey, or beef, to vary the recipe. White rice is a quick and easy accompaniment, but ideally serve with brown rice for extra nutrients and fiber.

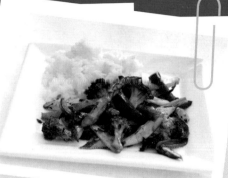

SERVES 2

- 1 tsp vegetable oil
- 1 fresh red chili, seeded and finely chopped
- 1 in (2.5 cm) piece of fresh ginger, cut into thin strips
- 1 garlic clove, finely chopped
- ½ bunch of scallions, cut into 2 in (5 cm) lengths
- ½ red bell pepper, seeded and sliced
- 5 oz (150 g) broccoli, cut into florets
- ½ bunch of thin asparagus, halved
- 1 tsp granulated sugar
- sea salt and ground black pepper
- ½ handful of fresh mint leaves

1. Heat the oil in a wok. Add the chili and ginger, and toss for a few seconds.

2. Add the scallions and garlic. Stir-fry for 5 minutes until shiny. Add the bell pepper and stir-fry for a few minutes.

3. Add the broccoli, and stir-fry for a few minutes more, before adding the asparagus. Continue stir-frying for 1–2 minutes. Sprinkle in the sugar, season well, and stir-fry for a few seconds to dissolve the sugar. Remove from the heat and stir in the mint.

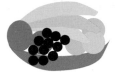

Healthy snacks

Eating little and often can help to reduce the symptoms of nausea, alleviate hunger, and give you an energy boost. Ideally, try to eat something containing protein to regulate your blood sugar.

• Chop up fresh vegetables such as carrots, peppers, and cucumber for crunchy crudités. Sugarsnap peas are delicious, too.

• Make hummus, guacamole, and salsa. Eat with strips of pita bread, crudités, or rice cakes. An easy way to get a little extra protein.

• Bake a batch of oat bars and add some seeds or dried fruit. The oats, seeds, and fruit will give you useful energy.

• Buy a variety of fruit, such as melon, mango, raspberries, and kiwi. Make up a fresh fruit salad and help yourself when you need to. Add yogurt for protein.

• Choose whole-grain bread wraps and rolls. Fill with egg salad, roasted chicken, or cheese.

• A handful of nuts and seeds is packed with protein and fiber.

• A small square of 70 percent dark chocolate contains nutrients and can help boost energy.

DID YOU KNOW?

DRINKING WARM MILK before bedtime can help you sleep and can stop you from waking up from hunger.

70% COCOA CONTENT CHOCOLATE IS A GREAT MOOD-BOOSTER.

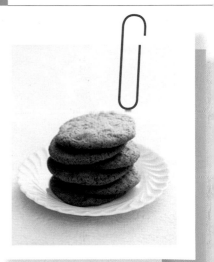

Ginger cookies

MAKES 24–30 COOKIES

8 tbsp butter, at room temperature
1 cup brown sugar (packed)
1 tbsp syrup from a jar of stem ginger
1 large egg
2 cups all-purpose flour
1 heaping tbsp ground ginger
2 tsp baking soda
¼ tsp salt
3 pieces stem ginger in syrup, drained and finely chopped

1. Preheat the oven to 350° F (180° C). Line two baking sheets with parchment paper. Beat the butter, sugar, and syrup with the mixer until creamy. Beat in the egg. In a separate bowl, combine the flour, ground ginger, baking soda, and salt. Whisk to blend.

2. Add this to the butter mixture, then mix in the stem ginger. Roll the dough into walnut-size balls. Place on the baking sheets and flatten slightly. Bake for 12–15 minutes or until golden. Transfer to a wire rack to cool.

Variation

If you can't find stem ginger in your local store, omit the ginger and syrup when making these cookies and use 1 tablespoon of molasses instead. Accompany your cookies with fresh fruit, such as strawberries, sliced mango, or blueberries.

Enjoying a night out

Eating in restaurants can become a bit of challenge when you're pregnant, so here are some hints and tips on which foods you can still enjoy and which you should avoid for a short while.

Main course

✔ Shellfish is safe to eat as long as it is cooked. Tuna is fine, but only in moderation since it contains mercury: no more than 6oz per week total of tuna steak or canned albacore tuna.

✘ Smoked salmon should be avoided.

✘ Game meat, such as venison, rabbit, and pheasant, is best avoided since it may contain lead shot.

✘ Shark, swordfish, and marlin due to high levels of mercury.

✘ Liver and pâtés.

✘ Avoid rare and undercooked meat—check that burgers are cooked.

✘ "Homemade" mayonnaise, hollandaise, and béarnaise sauces contain raw egg, so avoid them.

Cheeseboard

✔ Hard cheeses, such as Cheddar Edam, Emmental, Gouda, Gruyère, Jarlsberg, and Parmesan are fine.

✔ Stilton contains blue mould but is safe because it is pasteurized. If concerned, only eat it when cooked.

✔ Cottage cheese, mozzarella, feta, cream cheese, paneer, ricotta, and halloumi are fine, as long as they are pasteurized.

✘ Mold-ripened cheeses, such as Brie, Camembert, and soft, blue-veined cheese (such as Danish blue, Gorgonzola, and Roquefort).

✘ Goat cheese is best avoided if uncooked, such as in salad, but fine when cooked, such as in a baked quiche.

CAFFEINE?

It's fine to keep enjoying coffee and tea if you are pregnant, but you are advised to limit your intake of caffeine to 200 mg per day. Some large-sized coffees sold in cafés contain more than 300 mg in one cup, so be vigilant. Remember, too, that caffeine may lurk in other drinks (see right).

Measuring caffeine

8 fl oz filter coffee = 180 mg

"energy" drink = 80 mg

12 fl oz cappuccino = 75 mg

large cup of tea = 75 mg

hot chocolate = 70 mg

can of cola = 40 mg

Desserts

✔ Cooked desserts or desserts containing pasteurized cream.

✔ Fresh fruit, if washed or peeled.

✔ Processed soft ice cream.

✔ Honey; all types.

✗ Homemade ice cream, mousse, tiramisu, and soft meringue should be avoided because they contain raw eggs. Hard meringue is fine because the egg white is cooked.

✗ Uncooked cheesecakes should be avoided since they are made with raw eggs, but cooked ones are fine.

✗ Pastry dough contains raw eggs so make sure it's thoroughly cooked.

Alcohol

Even if you're accustomed to a glass of wine with dinner, it is advisable to avoid alcohol during your pregnancy, and with good reason: alcohol has been linked to preventable birth defects and developmental disabilities, and it increases the risk of miscarriage and low birth weight.

SUSHI

Sushi made from cooked food is fine. Shrimp, crab, scallops, and eel are typically cooked. Vegetarian options are safe, including avocado and cucumber rolls. Don't eat raw fish during pregnancy; it may contain harmful bacteria.

ASSISTED DELIVERIES

When help is needed

It may not feature in your ideal birth plan, but roughly one in every eight women has an assisted birth, and the doctor will only suggest it when it is completely necessary. If your baby is in an awkward position, if there are concerns about his heart rate, or if you are simply too exhausted, this may be the best course of action.

What's available?

Assisted deliveries are performed either with forceps or a vacuum (see below)—these instruments connect with your baby's head and help to ease him out of the birth canal. You will be offered local pain relief.

Forceps

One of the most common methods for assisted birth, forceps are like a pair of tongs, or two large spoons, that are eased onto either side of your baby's head to allow the doctor to lift him out gently, or rotate him slightly while you are pushing. They have a high degree of success, but may cause some tearing, or you may be offered an episiotomy (a small surgical cut to gain access). Don't worry, everything will be repaired and will heal. Forceps will often leave marks on your baby's head, but these will fade.

Vacuum

This method works by attaching a plastic "cup," which acts as a suction device, to the top of the baby's head. The cup is connected to a tube that the doctor will pull on during a contraction to deliver the baby. A baby born via vacuum may

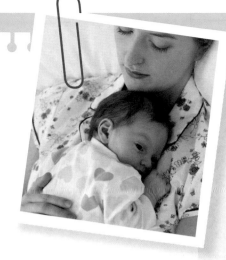

have a raised bump on his head (called a chignon), but it will disappear within 24–48 hours. The advantage of having a vacuum delivery is that the baby can still rotate automatically as he descends through the pelvis because the head has yet to "crown" (emerge).

Can I avoid an assisted delivery?

Unfortunately the short answer is no, not if your doctor has advised one. Assisted deliveries are only called into play when there is little chance of your baby being born safely without one. There are, however, ways you can reduce the likelihood of needing one—stay active as long as possible to keep labor progressing; eat snacks so your energy does not flag; and make use of gravity by trying upright positions.

Moving on

Ask to speak to your doctor if you have questions after the delivery or had a bad experience while in labor. Your doctor won't want you to be anxious, and can advise about the delivery interventions that were needed. You will recover quickly and there is an 80 percent chance you won't need intervention the next time around.

Natural remedies and medical choices

During labor, the body's naturally occurring painkiller, endorphins, reach the same level as those recorded in male endurance athletes at the peak of their treadmill workout. However, you might need a little bit more help on the day. Getting clued in now on your pain relief options for labor will help you feel prepared.

Nice and natural

There is an array of natural pain relief options that provide considerable benefits with no side effects.

Being immersed in warm water is soothing and supportive. The buoyancy frees movement and lifts pressure from the back and pelvis, while the warmth relaxes muscles and relieves tension (see pages 168–169).

A firm, sweeping back massage will release your natural, painkilling endorphins. However, on the day you may find touch unbearable.

A natural reaction to contractions can be shallow breathing, impeding the oxygen flow to the uterus and the release of oxytocin, the hormone that progresses labor. Controlled rhythmic breathing helps you focus, conserve energy for pushing, and releases tension, allowing your birthing muscles to work as intended.

Hypnobirthing combines breathing with positive thinking and visualization techniques to help you embrace the "surge" of each contraction that sweeps your baby along. Studies show that this technique can result in a shorter labor, fewer medical interventions, and a more positive birth experience.

You might want to try a TENS (transcutaneous electrical nerve stimulation) machine. This simple device uses electrical impulses to block pain messages, and can be effective during early labor. Pads are attached to your back so you can freely move around.

Drugs now please!

Labor is not an endurance test, so if it all gets to be too much, there are effective medical pain relief options that can help make your birthing experience easier to cope with.

Opioids are narcotics that attach themselves to receptors in the brain or nerves, blocking the transmission of pain. They may help you relax and have a more positive experience, but also may cause dizziness or nausea. They can affect your baby's breathing, so they aren't given close to delivery. Tranquilizers relieve anxiety, not pain,

"Heat relaxes muscles in labor— microwaveable heat packs mold to your body's contours, providing localized warmth."

but they can be helpful if you're very anxious about labor and delivery. They may make you sleepy and disoriented and make your baby sluggish.

For a total pain block, an epidural injection delivers local anesthesia into the space between the spinal cord and column, numbing the lower half of your body. It can slow progress, though, so you might be encouraged to forgo an epidural if delivery isn't far off.

A spinal block is a one-time shot of anesthetic in the spine. However, it can cause a drop in blood pressure and slow the baby's heart rate.

MEDICAL DIRECTORY

Pregnancy complications

Most pregnancy aches and pains are just a passing inconvenience and should clear up following delivery. However, some problems, where medical intervention may be required, are summarized here with possible symptoms and treatments. A high-risk pregnancy will always be closely monitored, so you will always be in safe hands.

Anemia (iron deficiency)

Having more plasma (the fluid element) in your blood means diluted red blood cells and less effective oxygen delivery. Symptoms include exhaustion and paleness, and affect a third of women in the third trimester. Iron supplements may be prescribed.

Carpal tunnel syndrome

Fluid retention in the wrists can result in pins and needles, and weakness in the thumb and fingers, for 50 percent of pregnant women. Wrist splints or steroid injections may be prescribed.

Chicken pox (varicella-zoster)

Up to 28 weeks, exposure to the varicella-zoster virus in the uterus can affect a baby's developing eyes, brain, limbs, bladder, or bowel; up to 36 weeks, a baby may get shingles as a toddler; after this, babies can be born with a severe form of the virus. The infection is transmitted to the mother by droplets spread during face-to-face contact. Ninety percent of women are immune. You should not get the chicken pox vaccine during pregnancy.

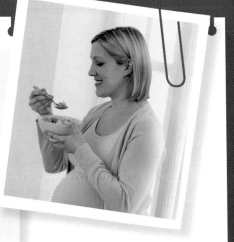

"If you eat healthily, you are less likely to suffer from illness during pregnancy."

Deep vein thrombosis (DVT)

Blood clots are more likely in pregnancy (when blood easily clots to prevent bleeding). Symptoms include pain and swelling in one leg, heel pain, and tender, warm skin. Treatment is required before a clot blocks a major blood vessel, and includes compression stockings, exercise, and anticoagulation drugs.

Ectopic pregnancy

In one percent of pregnancies, the fertilized egg implants in the fallopian tube, outside the uterine cavity, where it cannot grow. Symptoms from week six onward include severe lower abdominal and shoulder pain, and bleeding. If a doctor suspects an ectopic pregnancy, she will suggest an ultrasound. A ruptured tube is life-threatening, requiring immediate surgery or a laparoscopy.

Essential hypertension

Raised blood pressure is a common problem in pregnancy, especially after 20 weeks. It's a symptom of preeclampsia (see page 232) and linked to growth problems and premature birth. Lifestyle changes and certain medications may be prescribed and a 34-week ultrasound will check the baby's growth and amniotic fluid.

Fibroids

These are benign growths in the uterine muscle wall and can vary in size from a small pea to a large melon. They are more common in women of African and Caribbean descent. They can cause late miscarriage or premature labor. They usually shrink in size post-delivery and will be monitored throughout pregnancy.

Gestational diabetes mellitus

If insufficient insulin is produced to meet the extra needs of pregnancy, blood-glucose levels rise, usually after 24 weeks, risking early induction, diabetes, and metabolic syndrome for the mother, and birth injuries due to the size of the baby. Treatment includes healthy diet, exercise, and sometimes insulin injections.

Hyperemesis gravidarum

This most severe form of morning sickness affects less than one percent of pregnant women. Regular vomiting lasts for weeks, not days, leading to dehydration and sometimes liver problems. It usually resolves by 16–20 weeks. Rest and small, frequent meals help; in severe cases, anti-vomiting medication or steroid therapy is given.

Listeria

This is a food-borne bacteria that lurks in some soft cheeses, pâtés, and undercooked food; it can cause late miscarriage. Avoid the risk by cooking meat and fish thoroughly and avoiding soft cheeses (see pages 29 and 222), deli meats, and alfalfa sprouts.

> *"The majority of tests during pregnancy show that mom and baby are progressing well."*

Miscarriage

This occurs in 15 percent of pregnancies, although after 12 weeks of gestation it is uncommon and affects only one to two percent of women. The risk increases with maternal age. Miscarriage is a process, not a single event, so if you experience vaginal bleeding there are several possible outcomes. You may be referred to a specialist, but often no cause is found.

Obstetric cholestasis

Intense, persistent itching on the palms of the hands and soles of the feet extends up the limbs and is worse at night. This indicates a liver problem, causing a buildup of bile. If you experience these symptoms, consult your doctor. It affects less than one percent of women after 28 weeks, but is linked with premature delivery, bleeding, and fetal demise.

Parvovirus

Symptoms of parvovirus B19 are similar to those of German measles (rubella), but may be so mild they go unnoticed. It can cause late miscarriage, but in most cases pregnancies are followed by healthy live births.

Placenta previa

The 20-week ultrasound can diagnose a placenta attached low in the uterus, covering the cervix (the exit). Most move up by 32 weeks, but if not there is a risk of bleeding and a C-section may be required.

Preeclampsia

Severe preeclampsia affects 0.5 percent of women and requires immediate medical attention; untreated, it is life-threatening for mom and baby. Symptoms can include high blood pressure, protein in the urine, severe headaches, vision problems, vomiting, heartburn, rib pain, breathlessness, and sudden swelling of the hands, feet, and face. Medical management on medication is the cure, but it may mean early delivery.

Rubella

Catch German measles up to 12 weeks into pregnancy and the baby has a high risk of suffering cataracts, deafness, or heart and brain damage. If you had the MMR (measles, mumps, rubella) vaccine, you should be immune. It is not given during pregnancy.

Stillbirth and neonatal death

This occurs after 20 weeks into pregnancy. Before that, the loss of the fetus is considered a miscarriage. It may be due to a congenital abnormality, but 50 percent of stillbirths happen without warning. Stillbirth in labor is rare (1 in 1,000) and the overall risk in pregnancy has fallen dramatically due to improved maternal health and monitoring.

> *"Very common illnesses, such as colds and flu, are unlikely to cause harm."*

Stress incontinence

Women who have a vaginal delivery sometimes suffer from temporary urinary incontinence because the bladder neck has been stretched by the pressure of the baby's head passing through the birth canal. Kegel exercises will help.

Symphysis pubis dysfunction

Groin pain can be a sign of SPD, when hormones cause ligaments to relax. Symptoms can appear from week 12 onward and often feel like a muscle spasm. A "belly belt" will bring some relief. Ask for a referral to a physical therapist.

Yeast (candidiasis)

A yeast infection (white curdy discharge and itching) is more common in pregnancy and treatment is less effective, so a long course of antifungal cream may be prescribed. Loose cotton underwear and moisturizing with olive oil help; avoid scented soaps and bath gels.

Toxoplasmosis

This rare infection is transmitted through animal feces and soil, and can cause miscarriage and neurological damage during the first trimester. Wear gloves in the garden and don't empty the cat litter.

MATERNITY AND PATERNITY LEAVE

Time off work to take care of a new baby is available as official leave for moms and dads in most countries worldwide, but it can vary.

PAID LEAVE gives parents the time to provide great prenatal and postpartum care, allowing a greater sense of bonding. It also lowers accident rates in the work place.

A NEW DAD IN ESTONIA has to wait for three months after the birth of his baby before he is entitled to claim maternity benefit (there is no paternity cover). Only one parent can claim at a time, so if the father takes time off work, the mom has to return to employment.

ONLY FOUR COUNTRIES have no national law requiring paid time off for new parents—Papua New Guinea, Liberia, Swaziland, and the US.

IN GREECE, new dads are entitled to take only two days of paid paternity leave.

IN NORWAY,
"parental" leave is given,
which includes a quota of
10 weeks paternity leave for dads
that can't be transferred to mom;
in 2000, 90 percent of fathers
used their quota!

IN THE UK,
new mothers are entitled
to 52 weeks of maternity leave,
39 weeks of which are paid, though
this is set to change in the future.
Two weeks of paid paternity leave is also
available for dads. Many families choose
which parent stays at home according to
income—one in seven fathers is
currently a stay-at-home dad.

**ACCORDING
TO A US SURVEY**
in 2000, only 12 percent
of companies offered
paid maternity leave.

**IN THE
CZECH REPUBLIC
AND SLOVAKIA,** new mothers
can choose to stay at home on
maternity leave for up to three years
after each child's birth. However,
it is not common for fathers
to take any leave.

SWEDEN
provides working parents
with an entitlement of
16 months paid maternity leave
per child, receiving 80 percent
of their wages. The cost is
shared between the employer
and the state.

Pregnancy

acog.org
American Congress of Obstetricians and Gynecologists
Health information about pregnancy and its complications.

americanpregnancy.org
American Pregnancy Association
Information about all aspects of pregnancy.

babycenter.com
Information on conception, pregnancy, and birth, including free e-newsletters and forums.

hmhb.org
National Healthy Mothers, Healthy Babies Coalition
Information for pregnant women and new moms.

marchofdimes.com
Information about pregnancy, birth defects, premature birth, and babies.

womenshealth.gov/pregnancy
US Dept. of Health and Human Services, Office of Women's Health
Provides information, resources, and links for expectant moms.

smokefree.gov
provides practical help, advice, and support to smokers who want to stop.

thebump.com
Provides tools such as a due date calculator and pregnancy calendar apps, plus much more.

webmd.com
This family and pregnancy link provides a complete guide to raising a family, with expert advice from doctors and other health-care professionals.

whattoexpect.com
Pregnancy week by week and much more on this great website.

Labor and birth

birthcenters.org
American Association of Birth Centers
Find birth centers in your state.

bradleybirth.com
The Bradley Method of Natural Childbirth
Information about the husband-coached natural childbirth method.

childbirth.org
Information about pregnancy, labor, and birth, including cesarean sections.

dona.org
DONA International
Find a certified doula in your area.

hypnobirthing.com
Information and contact details for
HypnoBirthing classes.

lamaze.org
Lamaze International
Information about the Lamaze
approach to pregnancy and birth.

mana.org
Midwives Alliance of North America
Find a local midwife.

waterbirth.org
Waterbirth International
Learn about water births and
birth pools.

Breast-feeding

breastfeed.com
Information and advice for breast-
feeding moms, plus referrals to
lactation consultants and experts.

familybreastfeeding.org
Family Breastfeeding Association
Information and support for breast-
feeding moms, plus a helpline.

llli.org
La Leche League
Support for breast-feeding moms

naba-breastfeeding.org
National Alliance for Breastfeeding
Advocacy
Information and support about
breast-feeding.

uslcaonline.org
United States Lactation Consultant
Association. Find a lactation
consultant in your area.

Support groups

aafa.org
Asthma and Allergy Foundation
of America
Information and advice about
asthma, food allergies, and more.

acds.org
ACDS, Inc.
Support and information about
Down syndrome.

birthdefects.org
Birth Defects Research for Children
Information and support for parents
whose babies have birth defects.

cff.org
Cystic Fibrosis Foundation
Information about cystic fibrosis.

diabetes.org
American Diabetes Association
Information about gestational, type 1,
and type 2 diabetes.

epilepsyfoundation.org
Epilepsy Foundation Advice and support for people with epilepsy.

plida.org
Pregnancy Loss and Infant Death Alliance
Information and support for families who experience miscarriage or stillbirth.

nichcy.org
National Dissemination Center for Children with Disabilities
Information about disabilities in newborns, infants, babies, toddlers, and children.

nicuparentsupport.org
NICU Parent Support Site
Information and support for parents of babies in the NICU.

nmha.org/go/postpartum
Mental Health America
Provides information about postpartum depression and referrals for treatment.

www.postpartum.net
Postpartum Support International Support for women suffering from postpartum depression.

sbaa.org
Spina Bifida Association
Information and support for people with spina bifida.

shakenbaby.org
Shaken Baby Alliance
Information, prevention of, and support relating to shaken baby syndrome.

sicklecelldisease.org
Information and advice on sickle cell disease.

sids.org
American SIDS Institute
Information and support relating to sudden infant death syndrome.

stillbirthalliance.org
International Stillbirth Alliance
Information and research for parents who experience stillbirth.

ucp.org
United Cerebral Palsy. Information about and support for cerebral palsy.

Parenting

childcareaware.org
Office of Child Care, Administration for Children and Families. Learn about or find local child care resources.

fatherhood.gov
National Responsible Fatherhood
Clearinghouse
Information for new dads.

moms.meetup.com
Moms Meetup Group
Find moms in your local area.

nafcc.org
National Association for Family Child
Care. Information about child care
options, plus a searchable database
for local accredited care givers.

nationalsingleparent.org
National Single Parent Resource
Center. Advice, education, and
support for single parents.

nomotc.org
National Organization of Mothers
of Twins Clubs
Provides information and support for
families of twins, triplets, and more.

parentswithoutpartners.org
Parents Without Partners. Support
and advice for single-parent families.

General

aap.org
American Academy of Pediatrics
Health information about children.

cdc.gov
Centers for Disease Control
and Prevention. Health information
about pregnancy, children, and more.

cpsc.gov
Consumer Product Safety Commission
Find out about toy or crib recalls and
other safety issues.

nccam.nih.gov
National Center for Complementary
and Alternative Medicine
Information about acupuncture,
homeopathy, yoga, massage, and
other alternative therapies.

nhtsa.gov
National Highway Traffic Safety
Administration
Car seat safety information.

redcross.org
American Red Cross
Health, safety, and first-aid information.

safekids.org
Safe Kids Worldwide
Safety basics for newborns, babies,
and children.

**www.dol.gov/whd/fmla/index.
htm**
US Department of Labor, Family and
Medical Leave Act
Overview of the Family and Medical
Leave Act, including details about
eligibility and restrictions.

Phrase book
THE A–Z OF PREGNANCY AND CHILDBIRTH

Being pregnant can feel like being in a different country, speaking a different language as parts of your body you hardly knew existed are dropped into everyday conversation. This A–Z of pregnancy and childbirth terminology will help you speak the lingo in no time.

Albumin: Type of protein which, if found in your urine samples, may be a sign of preeclampsia (see page 232).

Alveoli: Tiny air sacs at the ends of the branches (bronchioles) of your baby's lungs. This is where oxygen is taken in and carbon dioxide passes out, back into your bloodstream.

Amniocentesis: Test to determine genetic abnormalities. A hollow needle is inserted through your abdomen into the amniotic sac, and a tiny amount of amniotic fluid is withdrawn for analysis. The test carries a risk of miscarriage.

Amnion: Protective membrane surrounding the sac of amniotic fluid.

Amniotic fluid: Clear, straw-colored fluid contained within a sac (the amnion). It surrounds your baby, cushioning him, hydrating him, and keeping him at the right temperature.

Apgar test: Your baby's first test! It's a method of evaluating a baby's health immediately after birth. There are five basic indicators: activity level, pulse, response to stimulation, appearance, and respiration. The baby is given a score of 0, 1, or 2 on each and the scores are added up to give an overall score out of 10.

Areola: Pink or brown area of skin around your nipple, which darkens during pregnancy. If you are breast-

"If you don't understand what is being said, ask your doctor—he or she is there to help."

feeding, your baby needs to latch onto the areola as well as the nipple, because it contains lots of little milk ducts that squirt out milk.

Birth canal: Passage from the cervix that your baby travels through in order to be born, once known as your vagina!

Blastocyst: Cluster of 100 cells that develops from the fertilized egg and implants itself into the lining of your uterus. The cells develop into all the different parts of your baby as well as the placenta.

Braxton Hicks contractions: Practice makes perfect and your uterus warms up with mild contractions as early as the second trimester; so-called because Dr. Braxton Hicks was the first person to describe them in 1872. They can cause confusion—is this labor or not?—but these contractions stop; real ones don't stop until your baby is born. If you aren't sure if these are the real thing, call your doctor.

Breech presentation: Baby is head-up and wants to come out bottom or feet first. Your doctor might try to turn the baby in the uterus, but if this is unsuccessful, you may be advised to have a C-section. It is possible for a baby to turn during contractions, and some are born in a breech position.

Cesarean section (C-section): When your baby is delivered through an incision in the abdominal and uterine walls. Cesareans can be elective (chosen) or emergency (unplanned but can be life-saving).

Cardiac output: Amount of blood your heart pumps around the body with each heartbeat—this goes into overdrive during pregnancy.

Cephalic position: When the baby is lying vertically in the uterus, head-down. An ideal position for labor.

Cervix: Lower portion of the uterus extending into the vagina. Your cervix

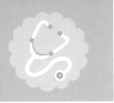

is sealed during pregnancy to protect the baby from invading bacteria, but when birth is imminent it gradually opens up to let the baby's head through.

Chorion: Outermost membrane around the embryo from which tiny fingers (villi) burrow into the wall of your uterus to tap into your blood circulation and grow the placenta.

Chromosomes: Cellular structures that contain genes.

Circadian rhythm: Internal clock that governs heart rate, breathing, temperature, and hormone levels over 24 hours. It takes your baby a while to figure out which activities are appropriate for day and night.

Colostrum: Thick, yellow liquid secreted by your breasts shortly before and a few days after childbirth, before your milk comes in. It's incredibly rich in nutrients and antibodies and gives breast-fed babies a great start.

Corpus luteum: Translates as "yellow body." This is what's left of the ovary follicle that released the egg that was fertilized. It pumps out progesterone to keep the embryo embedded until the placenta takes over.

Crowning: Point in labor when the head of the baby is seen at the vaginal opening. Get ready to meet your baby!

Dilation: Gradual opening of the cervix during the first "latent" stage of labor. Your doctor will check how dilated your cervix is—10cm is the target, when your baby can start moving down the birth canal. Then you can begin pushing.

Doppler: A device for listening to a baby's heart or blood flow through uterine arteries, based on ultrasound.

Edema: Swelling caused by water retention and blood pooling in your lower body. In rare cases this can be a sign of preeclampsia, so any puffiness should be mentioned to your doctor.

"Approximately 80 percent of infants are born with some form of birthmark."

Engaged: When your baby has moved down and two-fifths of his head is in position above your pelvic bone. Usually a sign that labor is imminent.

Engorgement: When your breasts are so full of milk they get hard, hot, and feel like they might explode. This happens when your milk comes in, usually between days two and six post birth. Feeding brings instant relief.

Episiotomy: Cut made in the perineum and wall of the vagina during childbirth to make more space for baby to be born. Surgery is required to repair the cut.

Estrogen: Hormone, levels of which rise rapidly in the first weeks of pregnancy, which thickens the lining of the uterus, swelling breasts, and keeps hair and nails in a growth phase.

Fontanelle: Gaps where the three bones of a baby's skull meet. The space allows the bones to slide over each other as the skull compresses on its journey through the birth canal.

Human placental lactogen (hPL): Similar to a growth hormone, hPL modifies a pregnant woman's metabolic state to supply sufficient energy to her growing baby.

Lanugo: Fine layer of fluffy hair that covers your baby from about 20 weeks; it falls out by your due date.

Linea nigra: Dark line that develops between your pubic bone and navel, thanks to increased numbers of pigment-bearing cells.

Lochia: Post-birth discharge, like a period, made up of blood, mucus, tissue, and clots. You will need maternity pads.

Meconium: Buildup of green-black waste in your baby's intestine that emerges as the first stool. Very sticky!

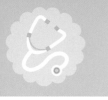

Melasma: Dark, uneven patches of skin on your cheeks, forehead, nose, and chin. Sunbathing makes it worse.

Montgomery's tubercles: Enlarged sebaceous glands around your areola producing antibacterial oil to keep your skin clean and smooth.

Oxytocin: Hormone that triggers the uterus to start contracting in the first stage of labor. If you are very overdue, you may be given an extra dose of synthetic oxytocin via an IV.

Perineum: Area between the opening of your vagina and anus. You contract and release the sling-shaped muscles here when you do pelvic-floor exercises (also known as Kegel exercises). Helps with bladder control.

Placenta: An organ that grows in your uterus to connect your baby to your bloodstream. It supplies your baby with oxygen and nutrients, in addition to removing waste.

Progesterone: Hormone that prepares uterus lining for implantation; also relaxes your ligaments and blood vessels.

Prolactin: Hormone that stimulates milk production.

Prostaglandin: Hormone that facilitates in the contraction of the uterus in labor.

Quickening: The first sensations of your baby moving. Generally felt for the first time at around 20 weeks.

Spider nevi: Tiny new veins noticeable on your cheeks, breasts, and legs, required to help your body disperse the extra heat your growing baby requires.

Startle reflex: Also known as the Moro reflex. Newborns are tested for this reflex to check that the nervous system is working. He will fling his arms outward, arch backward, lift his head, and cry.

Striae gravidarum: The official term for stretch marks. Caused by tiny tears in the

> *"Many cultures encourage a confinement period after birth, when mom rests and is taken care of."*

fibers of the dermis layer as skin expands quickly to accommodate your growing baby, breasts, and bottom. Think of them as well-earned stripes.

Surfactant: An important elasticating fluid that coats the walls of the alveoli. It is essential for lung expansion as your baby first breathes in air after birth.

Syntocinon: Synthetic form of oxytocin, given to induce or strengthen contractions if you are overdue.

Tear (in the perineum): Up to 90 percent of women experience a tear during delivery. First-degree tears in the skin heal naturally, second-degree tears extend into the muscle, requiring stitches. Third- and fourth-degree tears affect the anal canal or rectum and require surgery; this affects around 9 percent of women.

Transverse position: When a baby is lying sideways in the uterus, head on one side and bottom on the other.

Usually the baby will move of his own accord; however, if he remains transverse a C-section may be needed.

Ultrasound: A scan that produces your baby's first image! A handheld device (transducer) is applied to your abdomen by a sonographer and the sound waves visualize the baby on a screen. It is used to estimate your baby's due date and check for abnormalities.

Vernix caseosa: White, waxy coating that covers your baby from about 18 weeks while in the uterus.

INDEX

Acknowledgments

The authors and consultant on this book include an experienced midwife, as well as writers who specialize in pregnancy and birth. More importantly, they are all moms who have enjoyed happy and healthy pregnancies.

Our consultant

Judith Barac

Judith's belief that a woman's psychological well-being is of equal importance to physical well-being during pregnancy has led her through different areas of midwifery practice. Since 1997 Judith has consolidated her interests in the field of perinatal mental health; she is currently working as a midwife, a private psychotherapist, and a perinatal psychotherapist. Judith lives in London with her husband and youngest son.

Our team of writers

Shaoni Bhattacharya

Shaoni is a consultant for New Scientist magazine and has written for various newspapers and magazines, including Psychologies, and the weekly magazine for family doctors, Pulse. Shaoni has a degree in biology from University College London. She lives in London with her husband, son, and daughter.

Claire Cross

Claire is an editor and copywriter who has worked extensively in the field of health, pregnancy, and child development. During her career she has worked with a wide range of medical professionals. She also co-authored New Mother's Guide. Claire lives in London with her husband and son.

Elinor Duffy

Elinor has been a writer and editor of Dorling Kindersley books for over ten years, working closely with experts in their field. Elinor has three children, born in three different hospitals, and is the alumni of many a baby group! She lives on a farm in rural Hertfordshire with her family.

Kate Ling

Kate has an MA in Creative Writing, and is a regular Mumsnet blogger. She published her first e-book, Bad Roads, in 2012, and also writes, researches, and edits non-fiction and web content. She is married with two daughters.

Susannah Marriott

Susannah is a writer who specializes in pregnancy, baby care, and complementary health. In addition to writing over 20 books, her work has appeared in prominent magazines and newspapers, on BBC Radio 4, and on babyexpert.com, mumknowsbest.co.uk, and gather.com. Susannah lives in Cornwall with her husband and daughters.

Dorling Kindersley would also like to thank the following contributors: Proofreader: Angela Baynham and Indexer: Maria Lorimer.

Picture credits

Photography: Claire Cordier for the kind permission to reproduce her photographs: (p.10) Yew Hedge Maze at Longleat House, Wiltshire; (p.17) Bends Ahead road sign and empty road, Valley of Fire State Park, Nevada, USA; and Sadie Thomas for using her prenatal scan (p.59). All additional photographs © by Dorling Kindersley.

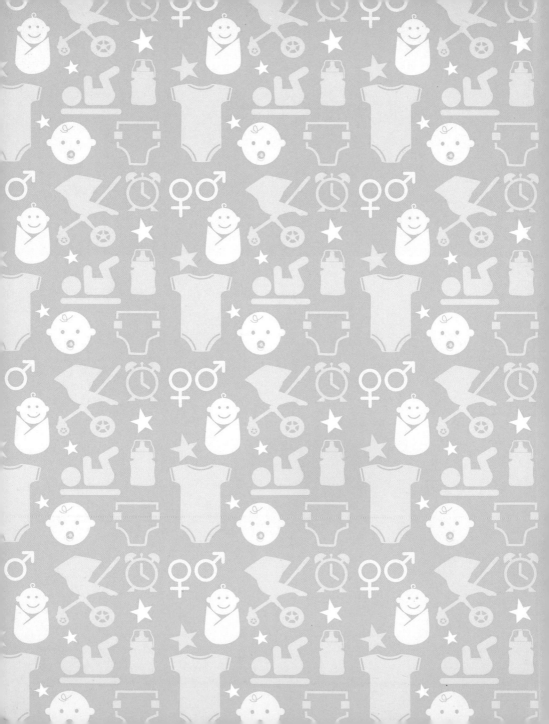